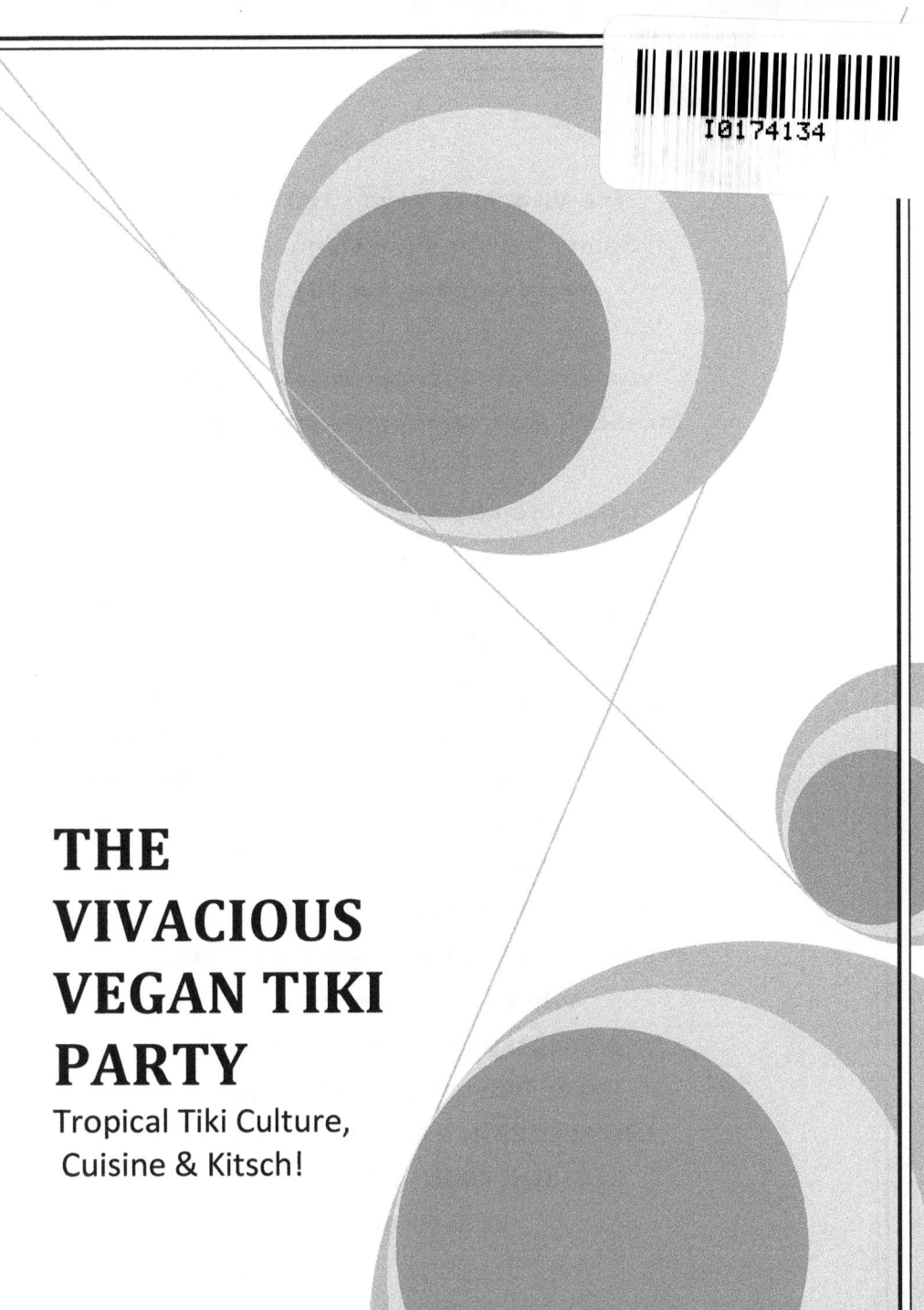

THE VIVACIOUS VEGAN TIKI PARTY

Tropical Tiki Culture, Cuisine & Kitsch!

Kathy Tennefoss

The Vivacious Vegan Tiki Party
Sunny Cabana Publishing, L.L.C.
New Orleans, LA 70115

www.sunnycabanapublishing.com
facebook.com/sunnycabanapublishing

Authored by Kathy Tennefoss

All Rights Reserved © 2012 by Kathy Tennefoss
No part of this book may be reproduced or transmitted in any form by any means, graphic, electronic, or mechanical, including photocopying, recording, taping, or by any information storage or retrieval system, without permission in writing from the publisher.
Published by Kathleen Tennefoss
Printed in the United States of America
Author: Kathy Tennefoss
Photography Kathy Tennefoss
Cover Illustrator Rin Kurhana
13-digit ISBN: 978-1-936874-22-4
10-digit ISBN: 1936874229
First Printing

This book is dedicated to my awesome friends and family or anyone who wants to add a bit of TIKI PARTY to their vegan diet! Who says that a vegan diet has to be boring or that you can't have guests over for a party? Your friends and family will be surprised when they try some of these vegan delights! Plus they are good for you and it helps the planet by eating a plant based vegan diet! Why wouldn't you want to share in the fun and through a vegan party!

Cover Design Kathy Tennefoss

Photos Kathy Tennefoss

Cover Illustrations by Rin Kurohana

First edition, 2012

Acknowledgements:

Thanks to everyone who has encouraged me to live my dream & to pass on the gift of health! And especially to my wonderful husband who inspires me every day and had to endure the countless trial recipe runs! (I really don't think he minded too much hee hee). I am extremely grateful to my friends and my family and I hope that this book helps others to eat healthy and to be active in their daily life!

If you have any suggestions, comments, or corrections please send me an email to sunnycabanapublishing@gmail.com or TheVivaciousVegan@gmail.com

Like us on facebook facebook.com/sunnycabanapublishing!

Facebook.com/thevivaciousvegan

www.SunnyCabanaPublishing.com

CONTENTS

Intro Page 7

Goods or Ingredients You May Need For Your Tiki Party Page 19

Tropical Quenchers Page 25

Boat Drinks Page 39

Appetizers Page 57

Main Courses Page 85

Desserts Page 103

Helpful Tiki Websites Page 119

Tiki Music Page 121

Hawaiian Sayings Page 127

Helpful Vegan Websites Page 129

Helpful Vegan Phone Apps Page 133

Vegan Schools Page 137

About the Author Page 141

Index Page 143

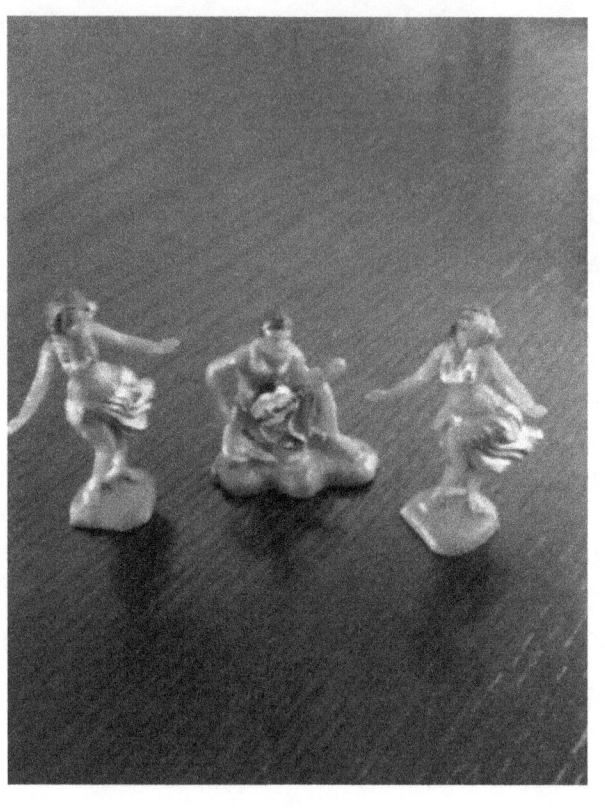

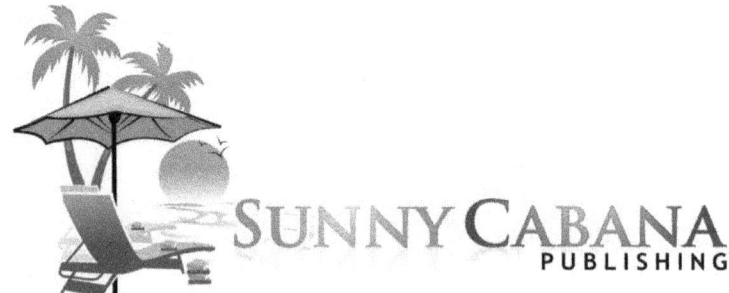

INTRO

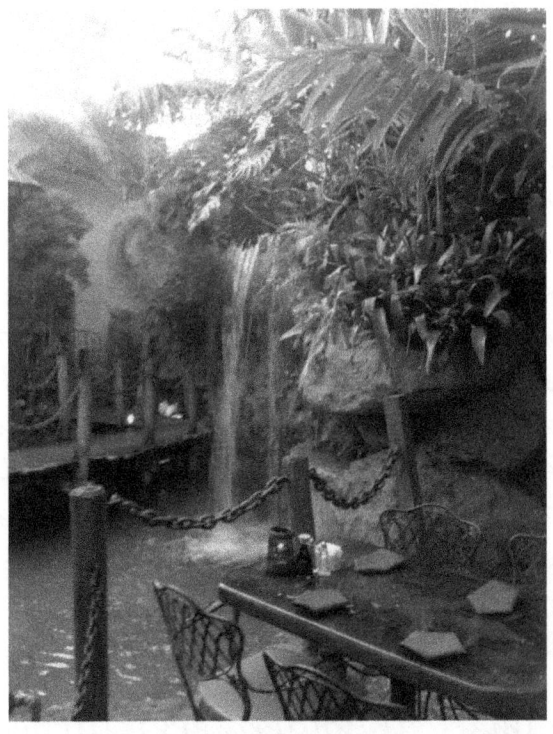

Aloha! I wanted to give you some information on how the Tiki Culture got started. America has had a tiki craze since Victor "Trader Vic" Bergeron spearheaded it in 1937 with the opening of his Polynesian themed hideaway in Hollywood, CA because he had traveled throughout the South Pacific. He changed his name to Donn Beach. Donn Beach is accredited to be the first restaurateur to mix flavored syrups with fresh fruit juice and rum! A couple of the drinks that he specialized are The Zombie & the Scorpion.

Today, tiki parties are a tribute to the '50's heyday with a fun, retro-cool style. The word "Tiki" conjures up images of beatnik fashion styles, smokey jazz lounges, flaming torches, fake palm trees, rattan furniture, rum drinks, and of course, wooden carved Tiki gods. Tiki parties are now seeing a resurgence, and can be given as a hip party alternative to celebrate just about any festive occasion, including holidays, birthdays, anniversaries, graduations, baby showers, and weddings.

When American soldergiers returned from World War II they brought stories and souvenirs from the South Pacific which also led to the fascination of the tiki culture in America. Plus with the onset of flights becoming cheaper there were more and more people traveling to Hawaii. Tiki parties just mean good clean fun! Everyone knows and understands the meaning of a "Tiki Party"! So grab your grass skirt and rum drink and shake your hips to your favorite rendition of tiny bubbles! (that was one of my grandma's favorite songs) I will never forget when my grandma took a trip to Hawaii and she brought all of us grand kids home grass skirts & puka shell necklaces! It was so cool! I think that's when I started to love the islands, the beach & the sand! As I grew older I grew to love the boat drinks too and thanks to my wonderful husband who absolutely loves Jimmy Buffet I have had a lot of exposure to great tropical music!

Tiki culture isn't just parties but it's also the music, hula girls, & fire throwers! (One of my favorite places to go is the Mai Kai in Fort Lauderdale, FL because they put on fire and hula shows and have a great Polynesian atmosphere oh and grand drinks!) There are so many hula companies who are teaching this technique to students! It's a great way to lose weight and have a great time!

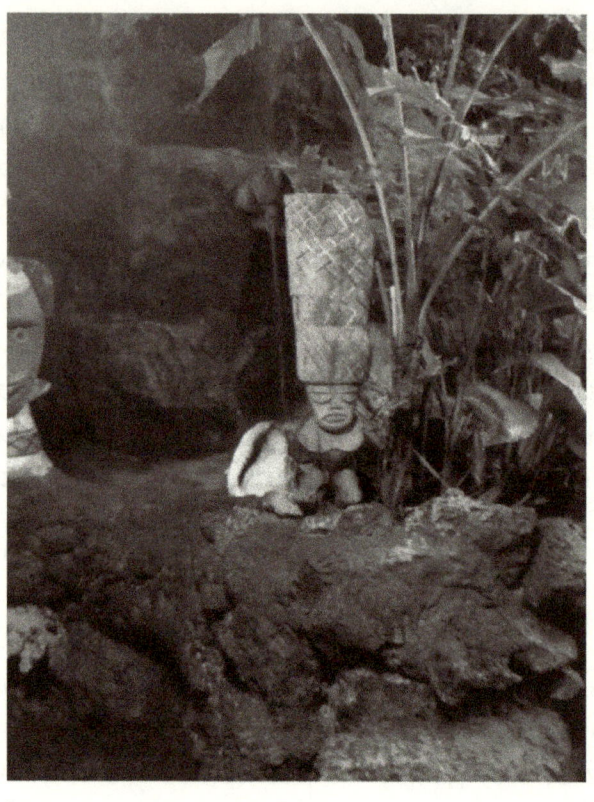

When it comes to tiki music the favorite instrument is the ukulele. The ukulele was most likely used by the Portuguese in the 18th century. The Portuguese immigrants worked in the sugar cane fields on the Hawaiian Islands which is how the ukulele started to become part of the tiki culture. They were sometimes called taro patch fiddlers because they were carried into the taro fields by the farm workers. I think I may get myself a uke and try to play! It just sounds like too much fun!

Tiki drinks usually conjures up great thoughts and good times (for most people depending on how many you drink hee hee). Most restaurants used to serve drinks in a tiki ceramic mug that you could take home with you and that sparked great interest in trying to collect them from all over the world! These drinks were usually made with rum and fruit like the Scorpion, 151 Swizzle, Planters Punch, Mai Tai, Zombie Punch, Fog Cutter, Saturn, Test Pilot, and many, many more!

What do all those tiki gods stand for? What do they mean? The tiki gods are used to decorate the Hawaiian and Polynesian homes. Tiki gods are also used to ward off evil spirits and to increase the odds of fertility by the owners of the gods. The four main tiki gods are Kane who is the god of sunlight, Ku is the god of war, Lono is the god of peace, wind, rains, fertility, & sports, and Kanaloa is the god of the ocean. There are some minor tiki gods which are Kauhuhu "The Shark God", Kaupe "The Cannibal Dog Man", Huakai "The Night Marchers" (the ghosts o ancient Hawaiian Warriors), Nanaue "The Shark Man", Lua-omilu "Land of the Dead, Maui, Pele Kanes daughter who is in charge of the lava flows. The tiki gods can be anywhere from 8 inches tall to 5 feet and can be used outdoors or indoors.

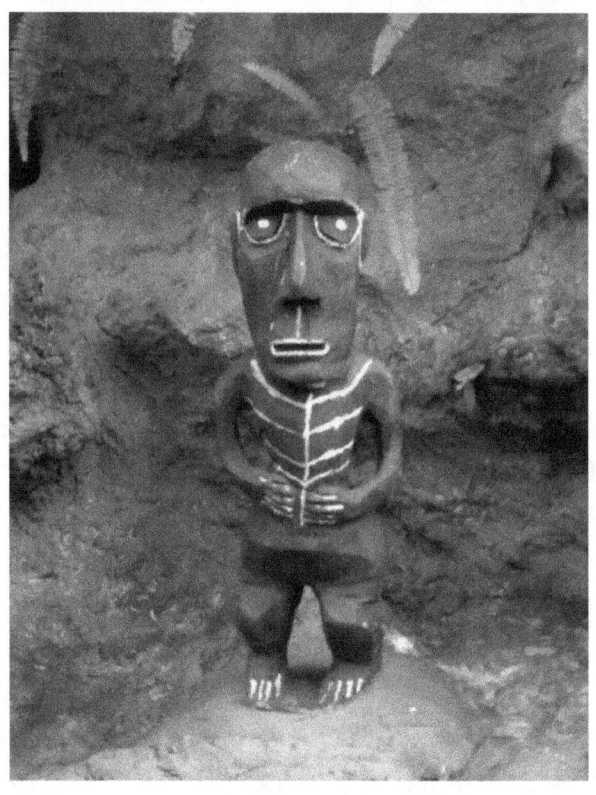

Other things that you should think about if you are throwing a tiki party is that is much better to have the party outside (preferably at the beach) because there are events that take place that would be better outside. One of the first things that you should do when you your guest arrive is to greet them with a Hawaiian leu. You can get these at most party stores or online at amazon.com. When you make out the invitations make sure to put what type of attire to wear. This should be beach clothing, flip flops, Hawaiian shirts, grass skirts, coconut tops, flowers in your hair, just fun things!

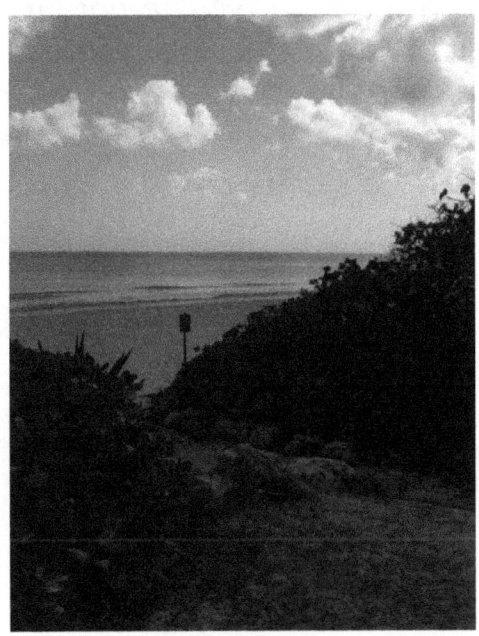

To make sure that your guests do not get bored make sure to have a few games for them. A cool one is musical beach towel where you play the music and everyone keeps moving around to a different towel and then stop the music and the person without a beach towel has to sit out the next round (make sure to take a towel away each time and also make sure you have enough beach towels for this). Another fun game is the limbo. This is where you have a piece of bamboo on a two stakes that you can lower each time everyone goes under the pole. However is left and does not move the pole with their body wins! You could also get really fancy and hire someone to come to your house that teaches hula lessons for everyone! That would be really cool.

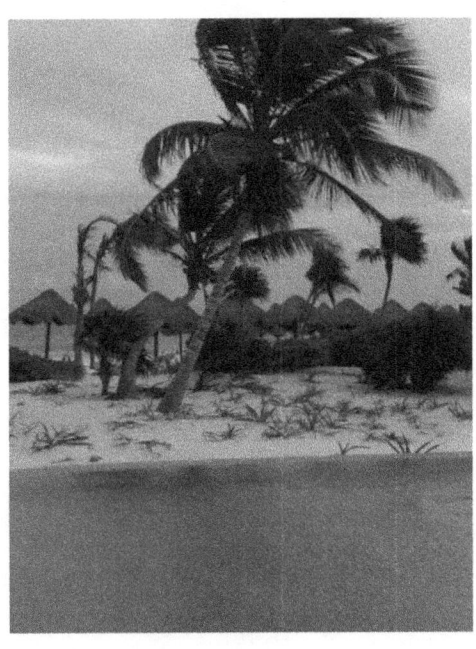

I want to bring the vegan diet to the tiki party! I want to change the thoughts that being vegan is just for hippies or natural beings! (Even though this is sometimes true. I greatly thank anyone who has put their health & diet first). Vegans are everywhere! They might be sitting next to you at the airport, doctors office you're shopping line or even your next door neighbor! Why not rejoice and invite everyone on your block to a vegan tiki

block party? You may be surprised who you will see!

These recipes are for having fun and entertaining! There are recipes for smoothies, appetizers, tropical cocktails, & main casserole dishes! Once your friends and families try these wonderful and fun recipes they will want to improve their health because they will enjoy the flavor and ease of the vegan recipes in this book! You will be doing them a favor without them even knowing it! Wouldn't it be nice to something for someone and have them not even know it! The biggest gift you can give anyone is the knowledge of health! This is the gift that keeps giving! PASS IT ON!

Follow us on facebook at:

Facebook.com/sunnycabanapublishing or

Facebook.com/thevivaciousvegn

www.SunnyCabanaPublishing.com

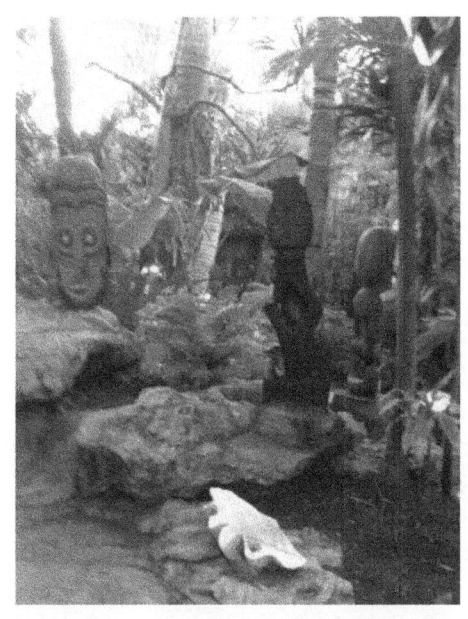

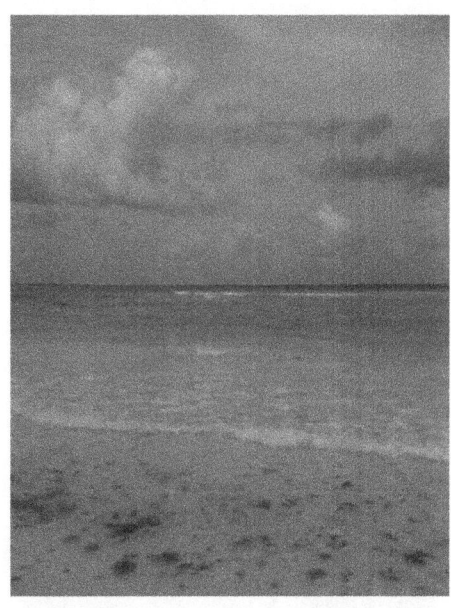

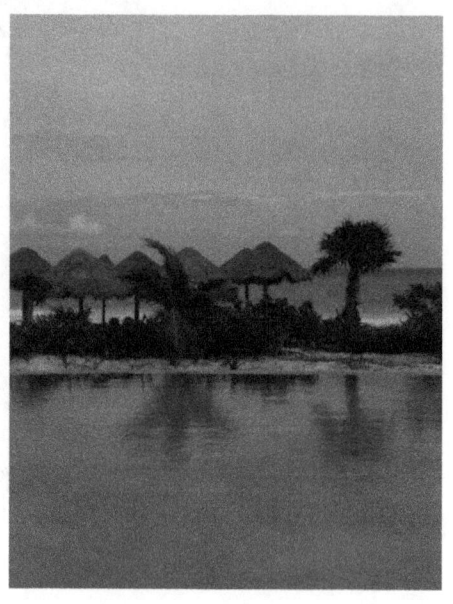

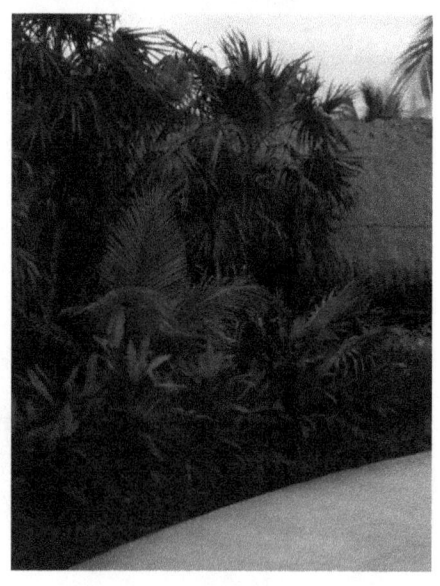

Goods or Ingredients That You May Need For Your Tiki Party!

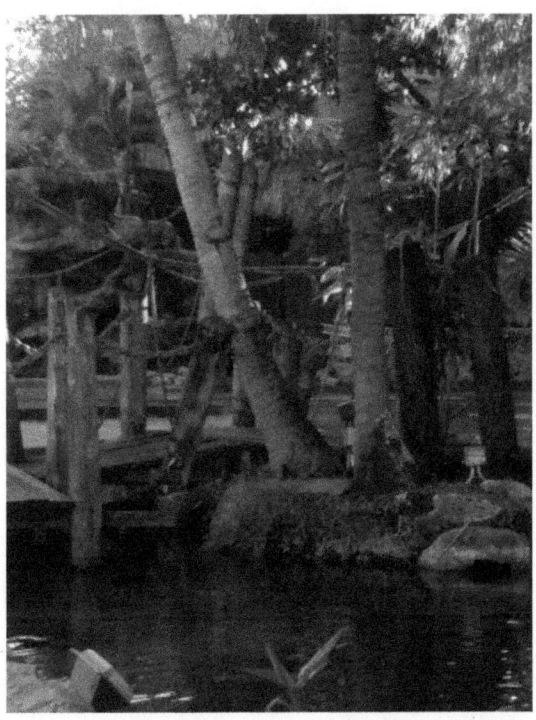

Tiki Mugs

Swizzles

Hurricane Glasses

Tropical Food & Drink Picks

Lais

Hawaiian Themed trays, plates, cups, napkins, tablecloths

Grass Skirts

Tiki Lights (if it's an outside tiki party)

Tiki Torches (also if it's an outside party)

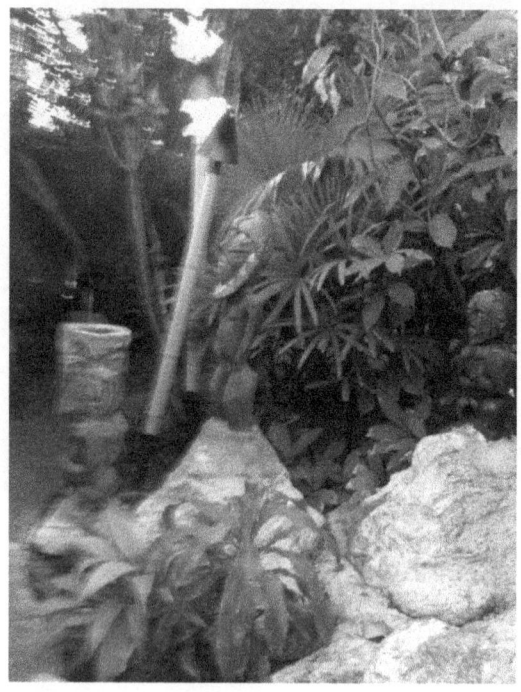

Tiki Gods (any sizes depending on if they are for outside or inside)

Tiki Music

Beach (if you have one by it would be great)

Surf Boards

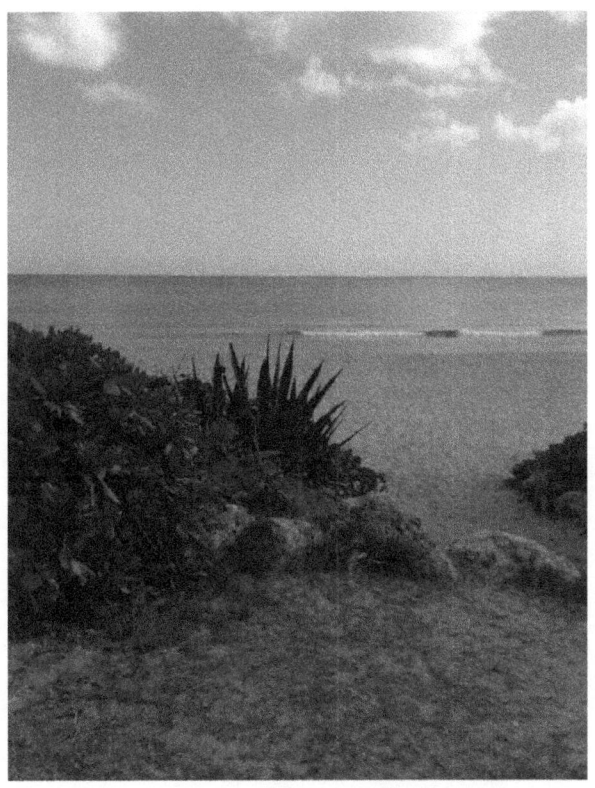

Food Supplies

Rum! Rum! Rum! Rum! Rum! Rum!

*Ice*Beer (for those who do not want to drink rum drinks)*Soda*Club Soda*Grenadine*Oranges *Orange Juice *Lots Of Pineapple *Pineapple Juice * Juice *Mint *Limes *Strawberries *Guava Juice* *Tropical Fruits (this will depend on the type of drinks you are making)*Coconut Milk *Coconut Flakes *Sesame Seeds*Tropical Juice This will also depend on what type of drinks you will make)*Tofu *Tempeh *Soy Curls *Gardeins *Veggie Burgers *Daiya Cheese* Veggies *Oats*Rice *Brown Sugar *Sugar *Agave Nectar *Powdered Sugar *Vegenaise *Vegan Whip * Tofutti Sour Cream *Tofutti Cream Cheese *Flour *Earth Balance *Braggs *Coffee *Macadamia Nuts *Cashews *Marachino Cherries *

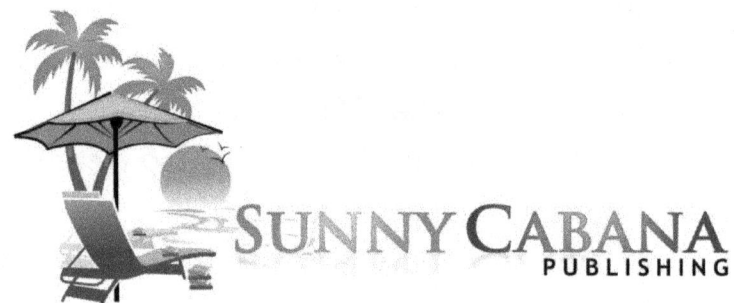

Tropical Quenchers

Pineapple Paradise Smoothie

Orange Cream Sickle

Strawberries & Cream

Papaya Tropical Madness

Key-Limeade

Citrus Teaser

Gimmie Guava

Crushing Passion Fruit

Pina Coolada

Sweet Papaya

Mango Orange Smoothie

Macadamia Milk

Mint Lime Crush

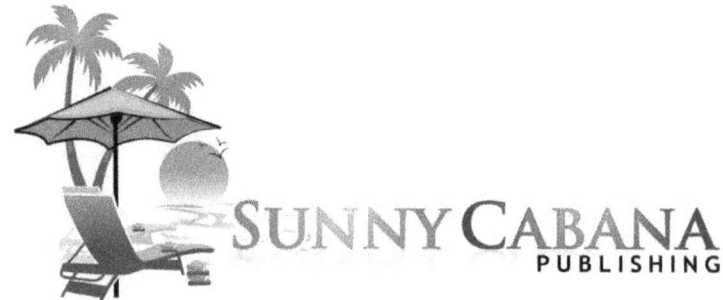

TROPICAL QUENCHERS

These thirst quenchers are great summer drinks or wonderful for your next tiki party! They are non alcoholic so even the kids can enjoy these delicious notorious drinks!

Pineapple Paradise Smoothie

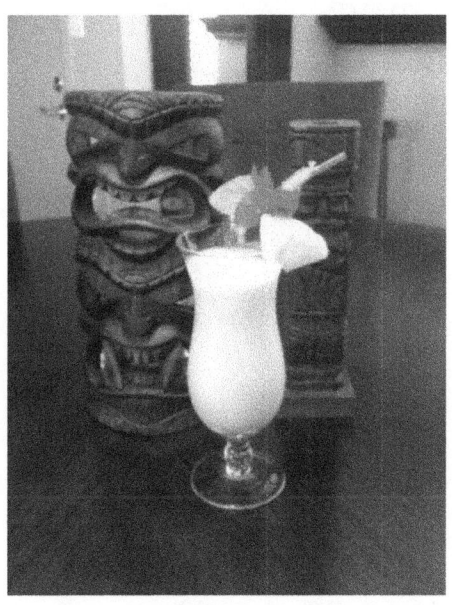

1 Cup Fresh Pineapple

2 Cup of Ice

1/2 Cup of Coconut milk

¼ Cup Pineapple Juice

A Few Sprigs of Mint

Take all ingredients and mix in a high speed blender and serve! You can save a bit of the mint or add extra for a garnish or a slice of pineapple, if you like! Nice and refreshing.

Orange Cream Sickle

2 Oranges (peeled and quartered)

1 Cup of Ice

1 Cup of Coconut Milk

¼ Cup of Orange Juice

Take all ingredients and mix in a high speed blender and serve in a chilled glass with a slice of orange as a garnish!

Strawberries & Cream

1 Cup of Frozen Strawberries

1 Cup of Ice

1/2 Cup of Coconut Milk

¼ Cup of Orange Juice

Mix all ingredients in a high speed blender and serve with a fresh strawberry as a garnish.

Papaya Tropical Madness

1 Cup Papaya

1 Cup of Ice

1/8 Cup of Lime Juice

½ Cup of Orange Juice

Mix all ingredients in a high speed blender and serve in a chilled glass with a slice of lime.

Key-Limeade

1 Cup of Key Lime Juice

1 ½ Cups of Ice

¼ Cup of Superfine Sugar

Grated skin of a lime

Take all ingredients and mix in a high speed blender and serve in a chilled glass with a slice of lime!

Citrus Teaser

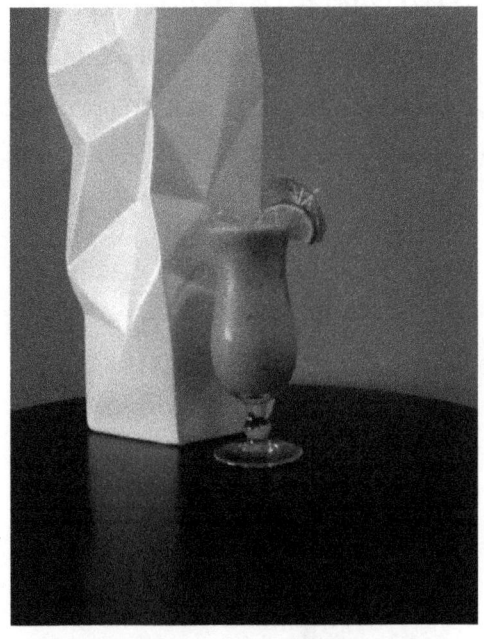

1 Orange Peeled and Quartered

2 Limes Peeled and Quartered

1 Lemon Peeled and Quartered

2 Cups of Ice

1/8 Cup of Mint sprigs

1 Tablespoon of Agave Nectar

1 Date (without the seed)

Mix all ingredients in a high speed blender and serve in a chilled glass with a slice of orange, lemon and lime as a garnish! If you do not like tart drinks then you may want to add a splash of simple syrup!

Gimmie Guava

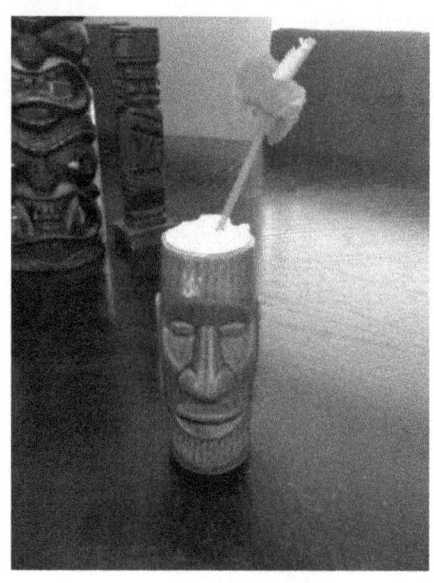

1/2 Cup Guava Juice

½ Cup Orange Juice

½ Cup Pineapple Juice

2 Cups of ice

Blend all ingredients in a high speed blender and serve in a chilled glass with a slice of pineapple for garnish.

Crushing Passion Fruit

½ Cup Guava Juice

½ Cup Orange Juice

½ Cup Passion Fruit juice

½ Cup Pineapple Juice

2 Cup of Ice

Blend all ingredients in a high speed blender and serve in a chilled glass with a slice of pineapple or slice of passion fruit.

Pina Coolada

1 Frozen Banana

1 Cup Fresh Pineapple

1 Cup of Coconut Milk

1 Cup of Ice

Mix all ingredients in a high speed blender and serve in a chilled glass with a slice of pineapple for garnish!

Sweet Papaya

1 Cup of Fresh Papaya cut into pieces

3 Kiwis Peeled and Quartered

1 Cup of Ice

Blend all ingredients in a High speed blender and serve in a chilled glass with a slice of kiwi!

Mango Orange Smoothie

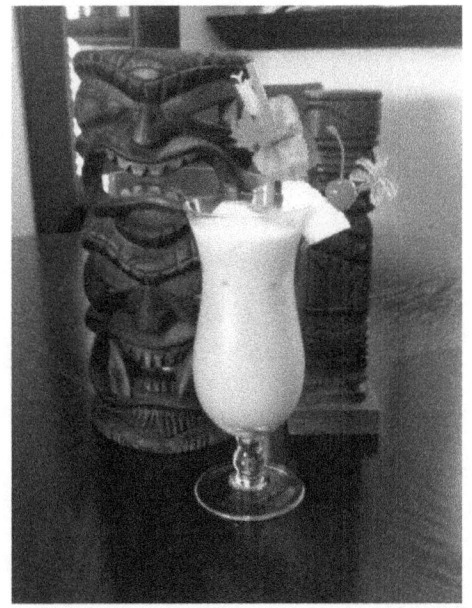

1 Cup Frozen Mango

1 Cup Orange Juice

1 Cup of Ice or a little less if you use frozen mangoes

Blend all ingredients in a high speed blender and serve in a chilled glass.

Macadamia Milk

1 Cup Raw Macadamia Nuts

3 Cups Purified Water

Soak the macadamia nuts for 4 hours. Next take the water and drain the macadamia nuts and blend with a high speed blender (Vita Mixer works best) until it is a milk consistency. You can use macadamia milk for your smoothies, rum drinks, appetizers, & even on some of your main dishes.

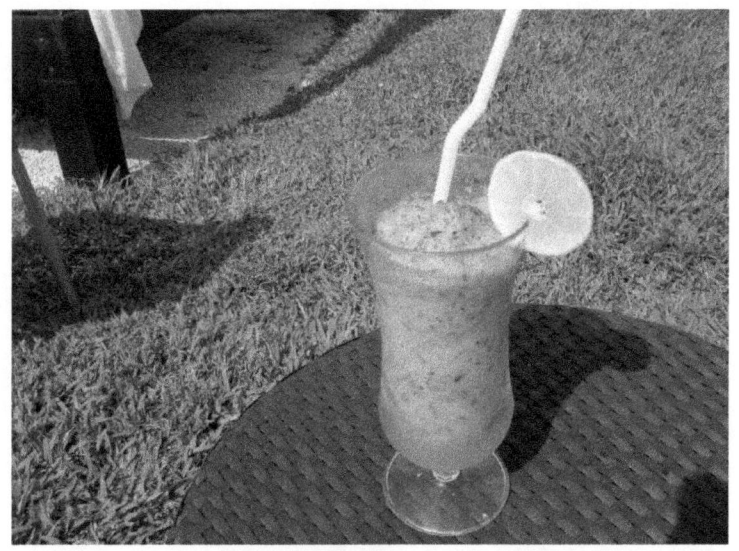

Mint Lime Crush

½ Cup Mint

1 Cup of Ice

½ Cup Lime Juice

1 Tablespoon of Simple Syrup

Blend all ingredients in a high speed blender and serve in a hurricane glass with a slice of lime and a sprig of mint!

Boat Drinks

Guava Coolada

Planters Punch

Scorpion

Mai Tai

Zombie

Rum Punch

Hawaiian Punch

Guava Sunrise

Lei Lani

Caribbean Coffee

Caribbean Cool

Banana Breeze

Rum Shot

Mango Daiquiri

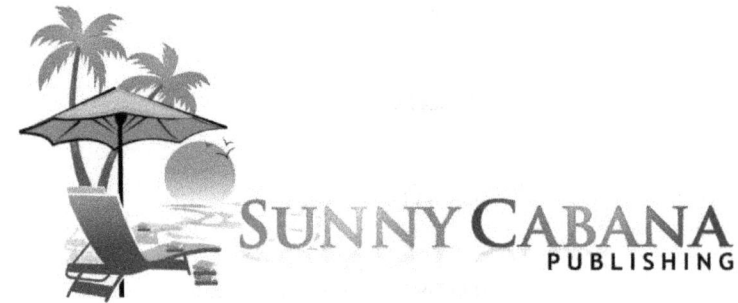

Boat Drinks

There are so many boat drinks made with rum! I tried to narrow it down to just the basic drinks but believe me there are so many more out there, ones with strange names, and some of them with familiar names, but either way it's all rum! It's much better to just pick a few drinks that you will make for your tiki party to make it easier on you that is unless you hire a bartender.

The picture is a typical glass/mug that most of these drinks would be served in. There are many tiki god glasses out there as well. Most people collect them so that everyone at their party will have a different one. Will these types of glasses there is no need for wine tags!

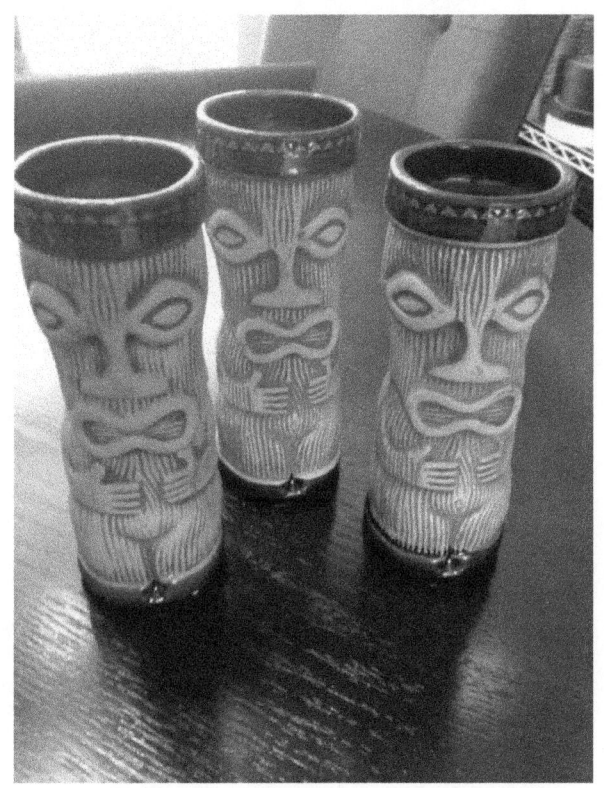

Guava Coolada

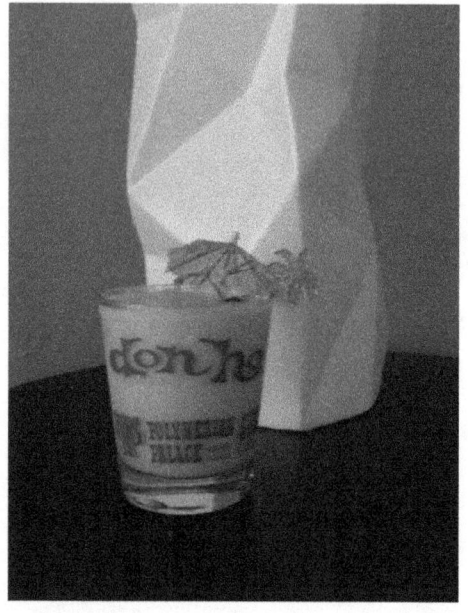

3 oz Dark Rum

3 Oz Guava Juice

1 oz Coconut Cream

1 Cup Ice

*Add a Grenadine Floater If You Like

Mix all ingredients in a high speed blender and serve in a chilled hurricane glass.

Planters Punch

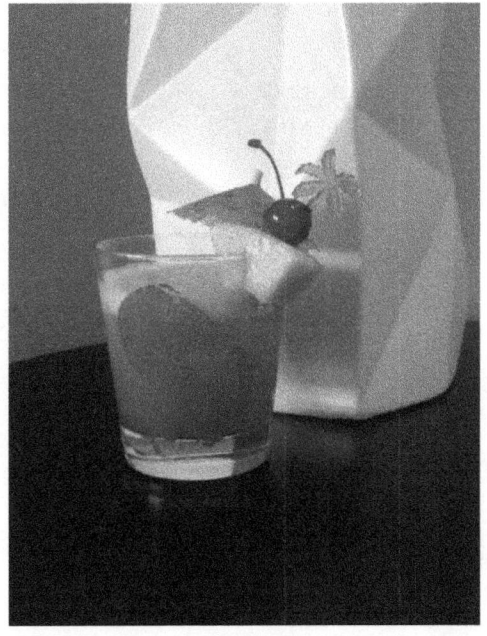

3 oz Dark Rum

1 oz Simple Syrup (equal parts sugar & water)

¾ oz Fresh Lime Juice

3 Dashes of Angostura Bitters

1 Cup Ice

Shake all ingredients in a shaker and serve in a chilled hurricane glass. Garnish with lime and maraschino cherry.

Scorpion

2 oz Orange Juice

1 ½ Oz Fresh Lemon Juice

½ oz Orgeat Syrup

2 oz Light Rum

1 oz Brandy

1 Cup crushed ice

Mix all ingredients in a high speed blender and serve in a chilled hurricane glass or a large tiki mug!

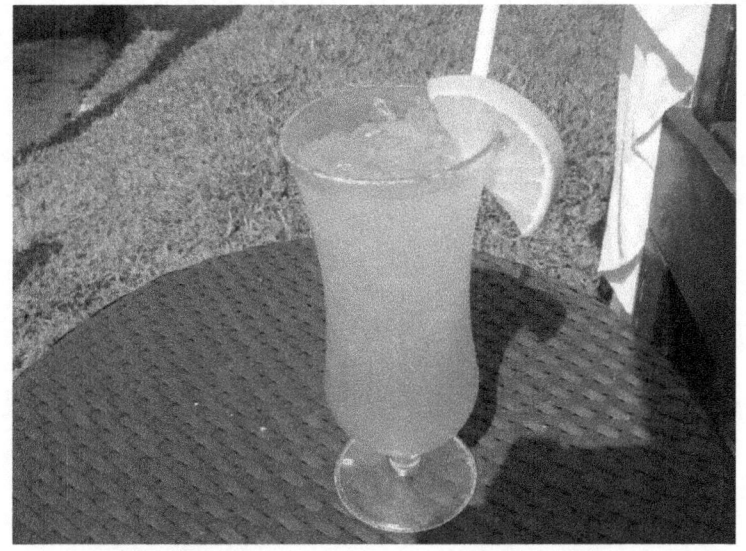

Mai Tai

3 oz Light Rum

3 oz Dark Rum

1 oz Orange Curacao

2 oz Pineapple Juice

2 oz Guava Juice

2 oz Lime Juice

1 oz Orgeat

Mix all ingredients in a shaker and then pour into hurricane glasses that are filled with ice and serve with pineapple slices.

Zombie

1 oz Pineapple Juice

1 oz Orange Juice

½ oz Apricot Brandy

1 teaspoon simple sugar

2 oz Light Rum

1 oz of Dark Rum

1 oz Lime Juice

1/2 Cup of Ice

Shake all ingredients in a shaker, strain ice, and serve in a chilled hurricane glass along with a slice of pineapple, mint, and a Cherry!

Rum Punch

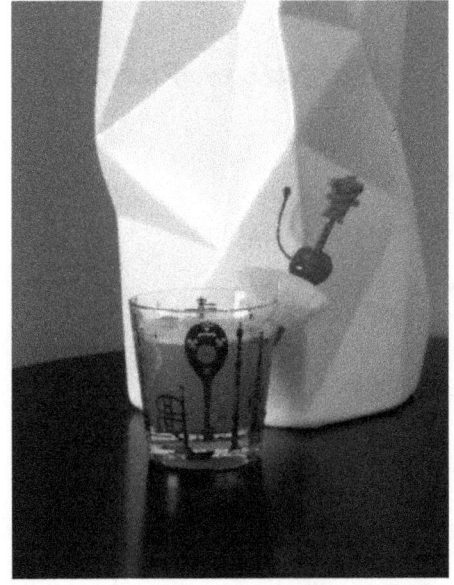

3 Oz of Dark Rum

2 oz of Guava Juice

1 Oz of Lime juice

1 Cup of ice

Shake all ingredients with a shaker and pour into your favorite glassware with a swizzle and slice of lime! You can either drain the ice or keep the ice to dilute the drink a bit.

Hawaiian Punch

1 Oz of Coconut Liquor

1 Oz of Guava Juice

1 Oz pineapple Juice

2 Oz of Rum (151 Proof)

Splash of grenadine Syrup

½ Cup of ice

Mix all ingredients except the grenadine in a shaker and pour into a hurricane glass and drizzle the grenadine on the top. Serve with a slice of pineapple and cherry!

Guava Sunrise

2 Oz of Guava Juice

3 Oz of Malibu Rum

Splash of Grenadine Syrup

1 Cup of ice

Mix all ingredients in a shaker except the grenadine and serve in a hurricane glass and drizzle grenadine syrup.

Lei Lani

3 Oz of Dark Rum

1 Oz Orange Juice

1 Oz Pineapple Juice

1 Oz Papaya Juice

½ Oz Lemon Juice

Splash of Grenadine Syrup

Splash of Soda Water

Mix all ingredients in a shaker and pour into a hurricane glass and add your splash of soda water. Serve with a slice of pineapple!

Caribbean Coffee

½ Cup Coffee

2 Oz Rum

1 Oz Amaretto

Splash of Simple Syrup

1 Cup of Ice

Mix all ingredients up in a shaker and serve in a big bowl like glass.

Caribbean Cool

3 Oz of Rum

1 Oz of Lime Juice

½ Cup of Soda

Mix ingredients except the soda in a shaker with a bit of ice and strain into a glass and fill the rest of the glass up with soda!

Banana Breeze

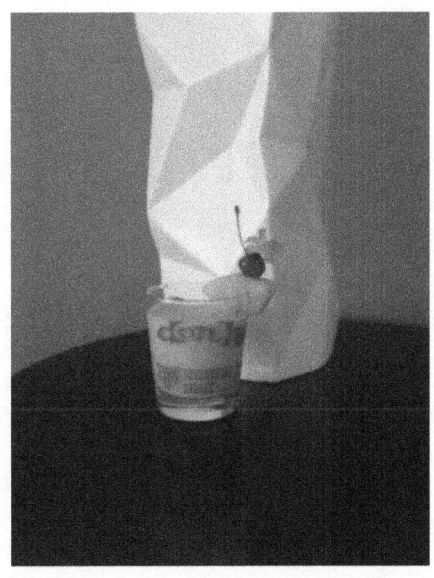

1 Banana

2 Oz Coconut Cream

1 Oz Almond milk

   1 Oz of Rum

1 Cup of Ice

*Add a Grenadine Floater If You Like

Blend all ingredients in a high speed blender and serve in a chilled glass!

Rum Shot

Shot of Rum

Grenadine Syrup

Put rum in a shot glass and top with grenadine!

Mango Daiquiri

2 Oz Dark Rum

1 Cup Frozen or Fresh Mango

1 Oz Curacao or Grand Marnier

1 Oz Sweet & Sour Mix

1 Cup of Ice

Blend all ingredients in a high speed blender and serve in a chilled daiquiri glass.

Appetizers

Taro Chips

Mango Salsa

Pineapple Salsa

Teriyaki Tofu

Ginger Tofu

Kahuka Corn Salsa

Macadamia Nut Tofu

Coconut Crusted Tofu

Sesame Tempeh

Macadamia Sauce

Grilled Pineapple Rings

Marinated Pineapple

Grilled Maui Onions

Tropical Salad

Watermelon or Pineapple Boats

Hawaiian Avocado Salad

Avocado Boats

Avocado Salad

Hawaiian Dip

Appetizers

Taro Chips

Taro means the star of the Pacific Rim!

2-4 Taro Roots (Depending upon how many people are at your party)

Oil for Frying

Salt and Pepper to taste

First boil a pan of water that is large enough to hold the taro root. Next place the taro root into the water and boil for around 40 minutes or until mostly tender but not falling apart. Remove from pan and let cool enough so that you can peel them. After you peel them slice into thin slices for frying (either length wise or round is fine depending on what you like). Once this is done heat your oil in a pan and fry the slices. Once they are done take them out of the pan and drain them on paper towels and salt and pepper them.

They should be eaten fairly soon after cooking so this is not a dish that you can prepare ahead of time.

Mango Salsa

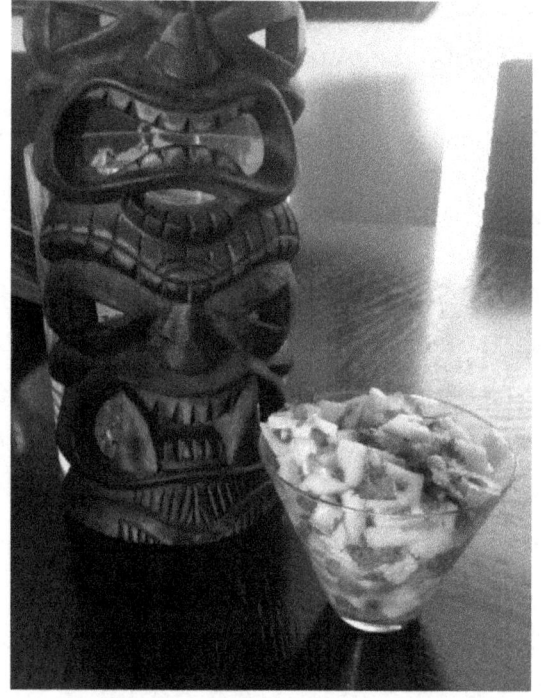

2 Mangos Peeled and Diced

1 Jalapeño Chopped Very Fine

½ Bunch of Cilantro Chopped

1 Garlic Shaved with a Micro Plane

1 Lime Squeezed

Salt and Pepper

1 Pinch of Cumin

Mix all ingredients in a bowl and garnish with taro chips. You can get taro chips in most stores these days or make your own if you have time.

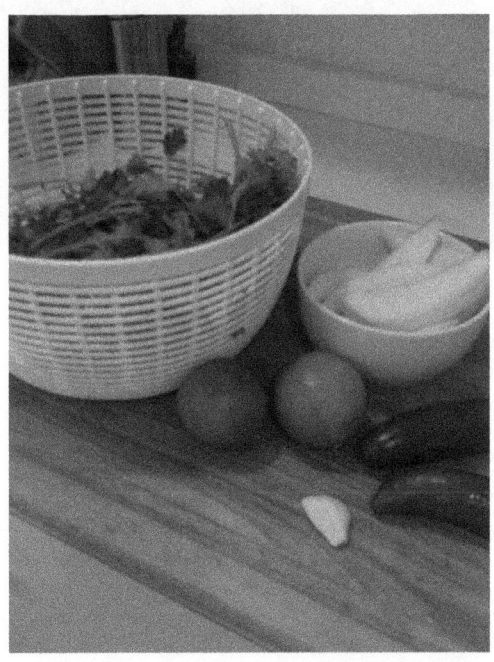

Pineapple Salsa

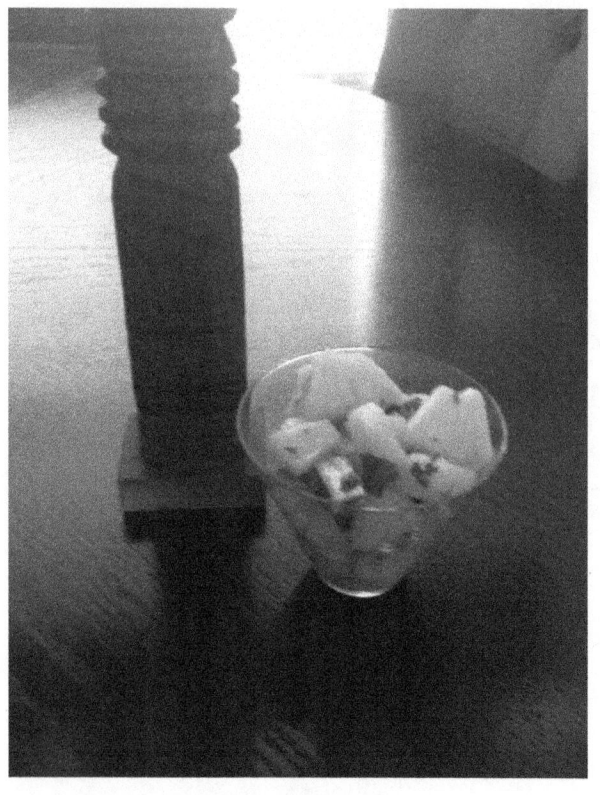

½ Pineapple Peeled and Cored

1 Jalapeño Chopped Very Fine

½ Bunch of Cilantro

1 Orange Squeezed or a couple teaspoons of orange juice

Small Piece of Grated Ginger

Salt and Pepper

Mix all ingredients in a bowl and top with your favorite grilled tofu!

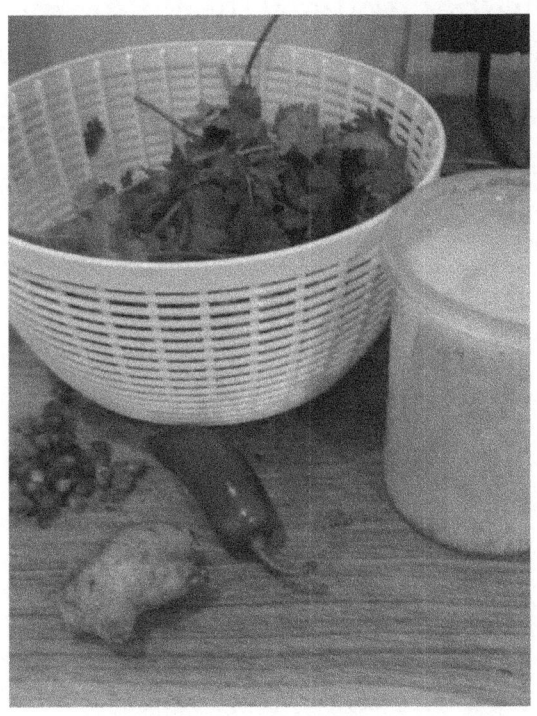

Teriyaki Tofu

1 Package of Extra Firm Tofu

½ Cup Teriyaki Sauce

First drain the tofu really well. Next slice the tofu into ½ inch slices and soak them in the teriyaki sauce for half hour. Then take the tofu and lay them flat on a broiler pan and turn after they are brown on one side. Serve with a side of teriyaki sauce for dipping.

Ginger Tofu

½ Cup Soy Sauce

1 Tablespoon of Agave Nectar

Large Piece of Ginger grated

1 Package of Extra Firm Tofu

Take the soy sauce, agave, and grated ginger and mix well. Take the tofu and drain and slice into ¼ inch slices and soak in the sauce. After soaking for half hour, broil both sides and serve.

Kahuka Corn Salsa

Fresh Corn Cut from the cob

1 Cup Pineapple Diced

½ Bunch of Cilantro

Pinch of Cumin

Pinch of Red Pepper Flakes

Salt and Pepper to taste

Take all ingredients and mix well and serve on top of grilled tofu or with taro chips.

Macadamia Nut Crusted Tofu

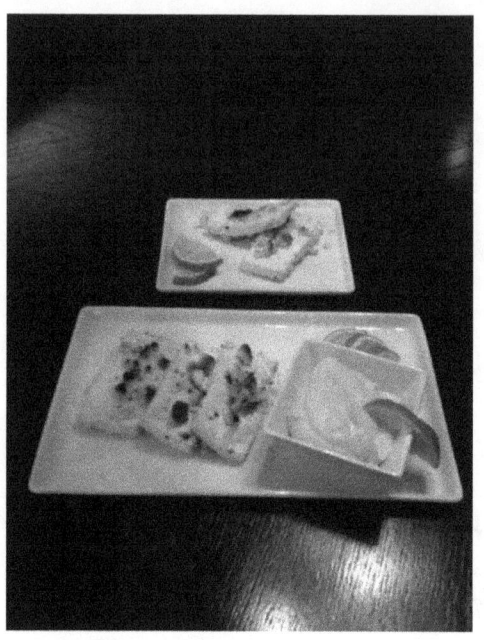

1 Package Extra Firm Tofu Drained

½ Cup Coconut Milk

3/4 Cup of Finely Chopped Macadamia Nuts

Salt & Pepper

A Bit of Flour

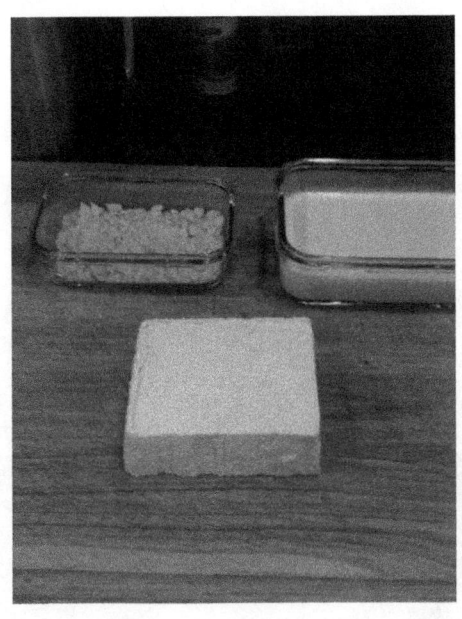

First make sure that the tofu is drained well. You can also wrap the tofu in a couple of paper towels to make sure the water is out. Take the paper towels off of the tofu and slice into ¼ inch thick slices. Now take the tofu slices and soak in the coconut milk, put flour on both sides of tofu, and coat with the macadamia nuts. Broil both sides of the tofu until crispy and serve with Macadamia sauce.

Coconut Crusted Tofu

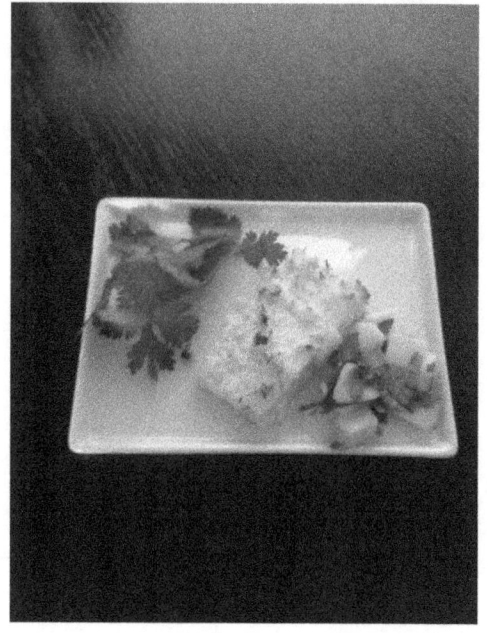

1 Package of Extra Firm Tofu Drained

½ Cup Dried Coconut

½ Cup Coconut Milk

*1 Tablespoon Soy Sauce

First make sure the tofu is drained well. Next take the tofu and slice into ¼ inch slices and soak in the coconut milk and then coat evenly with the dried coconut milk. Now take and broil the tofu on both sides until golden brown.

*You can also use Braggs Amino Acid instead of soy sauce I prefer this)

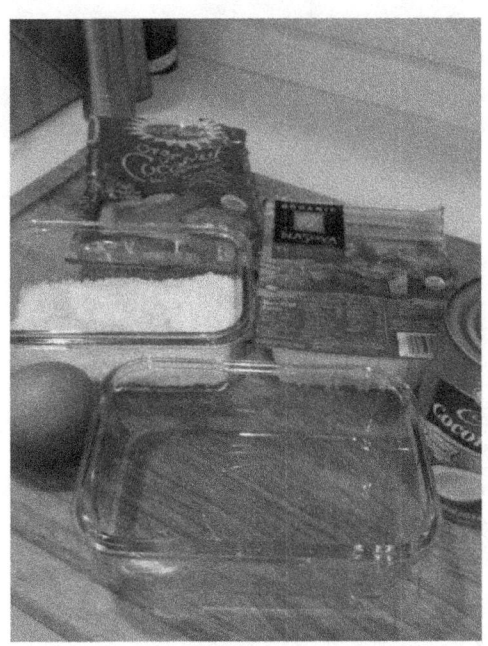

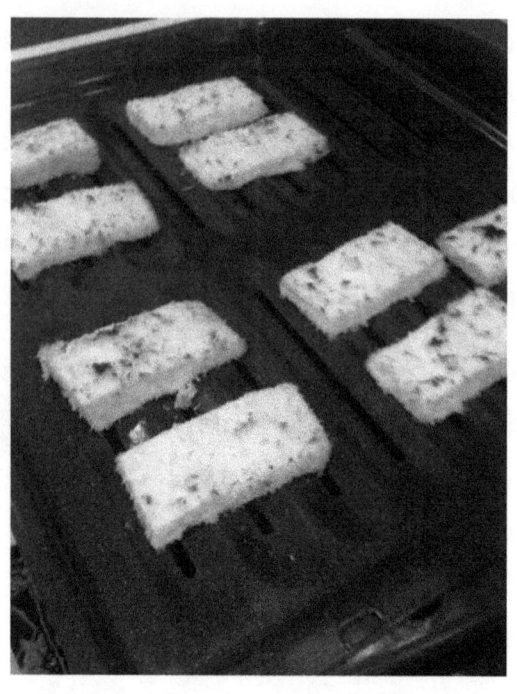

Sesame Encrusted Tempeh

1 Package of Any Flavor Tempeh

Dried black and yellow sesame seeds

½ Cup Teriyaki sauce

Cut the tempeh into bite size pieces and coat with the teriyaki sauce

Macadamia Sauce

1 Cup Raw Macadamia nuts (soaked for 4 hours)

¼ Cup Lime Juice

¼ Cup of the left over soaking water

½ Cup Coconut Milk

1 Tablespoon of Braggs

2 Tablespoon of Brown Rice Syrup

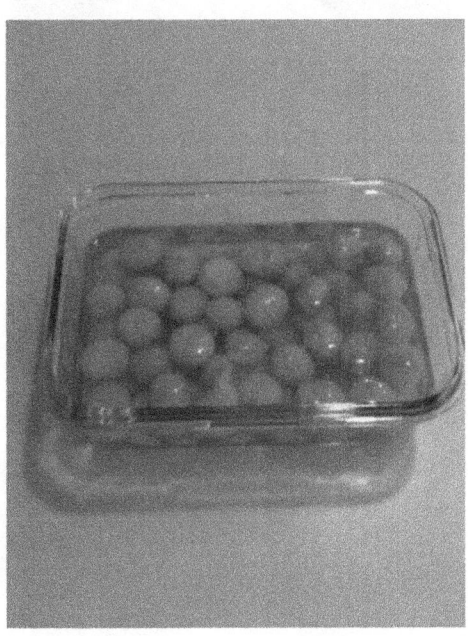

Drain the macadamia nuts and then take all of the other ingredients and blend in a high speed blender until smooth and serve with the macadamia nut crusted tofu or the coconut crusted tofu.

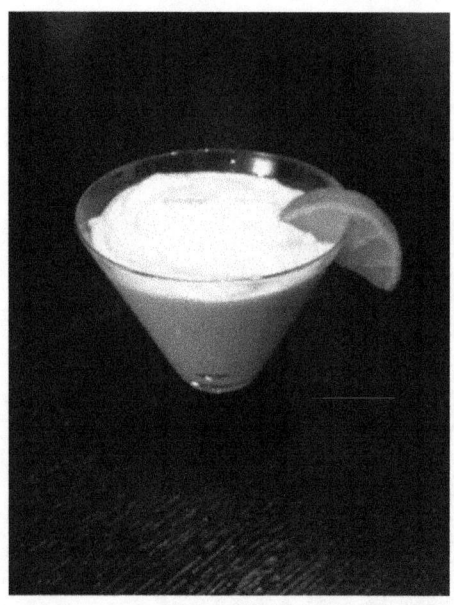

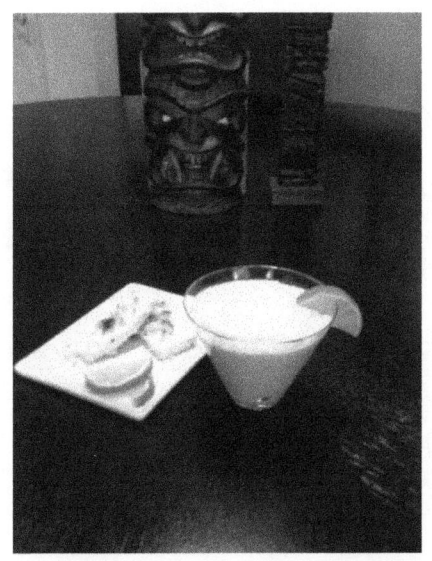

Grilled Pineapple Rings

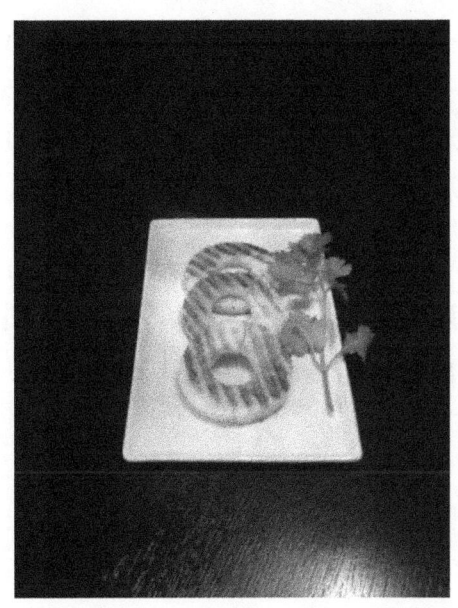

1 Ripe Pineapple

A bit of Macadamia Oil

Salt and Pepper for taste

*If you like it a bit spicier you can add a bit of red pepper flakes to the mixture (this is what I prefer)

First take and peel and core the pineapple and slice into rings. Next take and coat each ring front and back with the oil and salt and pepper and then grill on both sides till golden brown. You can also use the macadamia sauce as a garnish for this dish!

*Another great way to prepare this dish is to soak the pineapple in coconut milk and coconut flakes and grill! Yummy!

Marinated Pineapple

2-4 Cups of Fresh Pineapple cut into chunks (the amount you will need for the recipe is determined by how many people are coming to your party)

½ Cup Rum (this will also depend on the amount of people are coming over)

½ Cup Sugar

Sliced limes

First take the pineapple chunks and soak with the sugar and rum for 1-2 hours and them serve with your favorite sliced fruit and limes!

Grilled Maui Onions

2-3 Large Maui Onions

½ Cup Macadamia Oil or Olive Oil

¼ -1/2 Cup Soy Sauce

Salt and Pepper to taste

First peel the onions and then slice in think rings and marinate with the rest of the ingredients and then grill on both sides until golden brown!

Tropical Salad

1 Mango Peeled and Chopped Into Small Pieces

1 Papaya Peeled, Deseeded, and Chopped Into Small Pieces

1 Cucumber Peeled and Sliced Into Small Pieces

1 Maui Onion Peeled and Sliced Into Small Pieces

1 Bunch of Cilantro

2 Tablespoons of Olive Oil

1-2 Limes Squeezed

1 Clove of Garlic Minced

Salt And Pepper To Taste

Take the chopped fruit and toss with the olive oil, garlic, and fresh lime juice and serve!

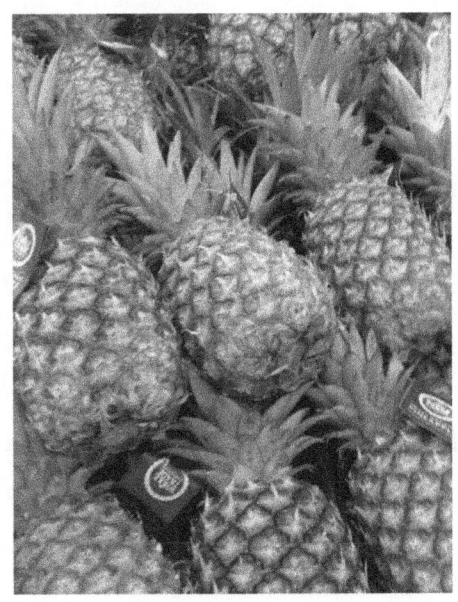

Watermelon or Pineapple Boats

These are great for a large party!

1 Large Watermelon

1 Pineapple

1 Large Quart of Strawberries

First take and but the watermelon and pineapple in half. Next take a melon baler and scoop the watermelon out into another bowl until all of the melon is gone. Next take and cut the pineapple out of its shell and try not to puncture the pineapple all the way through. Take the pineapple pieces and cut them into chunks. Take the strawberries and clean and wash them and cut them in half. Now take all the fruit and place it in the halves of watermelon and pineapple. These make a great display and taste great too!

Hawaiian Avocado Salsa

3-4 Avocados

3 Limes

2 Tablespoons of Olive Oil

1 Teaspoon of Cumin

1 Clove of Garlic minced

1 Large Cucumber

Peel and cut avocado and cucumber into small chunks and then toss with the rest of the ingredients and serve!

Avocado Boats

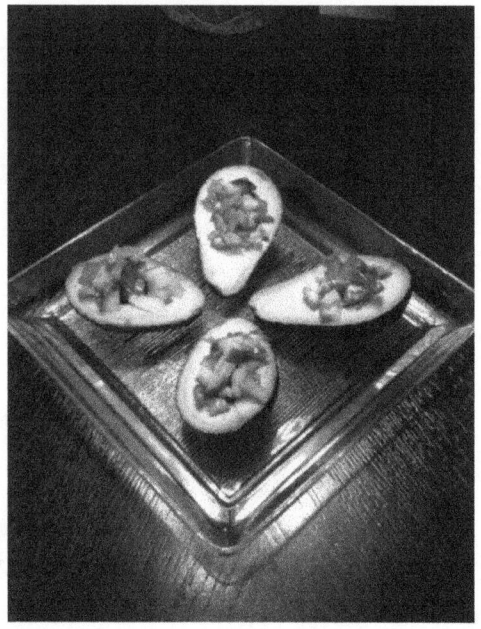

3-4 Avocados Cut In Half with the Seed Taken Out

1/4 Cup Lime Juice

1 Teaspoon Olive Oil

½ Each of Tri Colored Peppers Diced Really Small

1 Cucumber Diced small

¼ Cup Chopped Cilantro

Salt and Pepper

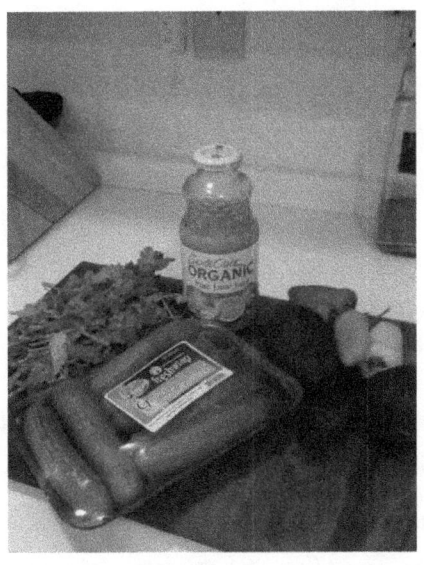

Take the red pepper and cucumber and toss with the lime juice and salt and pepper and scoop into the avocado and serve. You can do this with many ingredients! It has great presentation and is fun!

Avocado Salad

3 Avocados

4-5 Bunches of Endive

1 Papaya

1 Lime Squeezed

Champagne Vinegar

Salt And Pepper To Taste

First take and cut the avocados in half and take the seed out. Cut into small pieces and set aside. Next take the papaya and cut in half and take the seeds out and cut that into small pieces. Now take the lime, vinegar, olive oil, salt and pepper and mix in a separate bowl to make a dressing. Now take the endive and separate the leaves on a platter. Next take the avocado and papaya and mix together and place by spoonfuls in the endive and drizzle with the dressing! These are great finger appetizers!

Hawaiian Dip

¾ Cup Coconut Milk (you can use almond milk if you prefer)

½ Cup Tofutti Sour Cream

8 oz Pineapple with Its Juice

1 Tablespoon of Lime Juice & the Zest

1/3 Cup Toasted Coconut

1 Tablespoon of Powdered Sugar

Mix all ingredients in a bowl and chill for 1 hour and serve with bread, carrot sticks, or celery sticks!

Main Courses

Hawaiian Fried Rice

Hawaiian Soy Curls

Hawaiian Kabobs

Hawaiian Sweet Potatoes

Taro Root with Tempeh

BBQ Soy Curls

Tofu Hawaiian Stay

Grilled Eggplant

Grilled Gardeins

Hawaiian Gardeins with Pineapple

Hawaiian Gardeins

Hawaiian Rum Gardeins

Vegan Hawiian BBQ Burgers

Hawiian Macaroni Salad

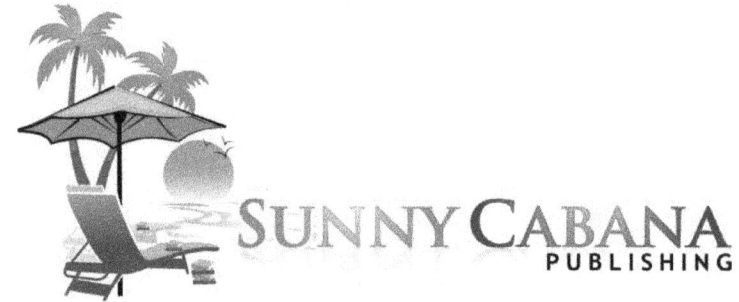

Main Courses

Hawaiian Fried Rice

This is one of the staples for any tiki party! You can omit the macadamia nuts if you like but I think they give this dish a great nutty flavor!

2 Cups Cooked Rice

1 Teaspoon of Sesame Oil

¼ Cup Diced Carrots

½ Cup Diced Pineapple

½ Cup Macadamia Nuts Chopped

2 Tablespoons of Soy Sauce

1 Cup Fried Tofu

Heat the oil in a wok like pan and then add the tofu so that it will get golden brown. Next add the carrots. After a couple more minutes add the rest of the ingredients until it is golden brown and serve! If it starts to stick don't add more sesame oil because the flavor will be too intense. You can add a bit of olive oil or vegetable oil if you need to.

Hawaiian Soy Curls

1 Package of Soy Curls (soak them for the required time first and then drain them)

2 Cups Pineapple cut into small chunks

3 Tablespoons of Soy Sauce

1/2-3/4 Cups of Teriyaki Sauce

Sliced Green Onion for Garnish

¼ Cup Cilantro

Once the soy curls are drained take the rest of the ingredients and mix together well and then bake at 350 degrees for 25 minutes and serve!

Hawaiian Kabobs

20 or so Button Mushrooms

20 Or So of Pineapple Chunks

20 Or So Small Cherry Tomatoes

20 Or So f Maui Onion Chunks

Marinated Tempeh or Soy Curls

Skewers Metal if you have them

Sauce:

¼ Cup Soy Sauce

½ Cup Pineapple Juice

1 Tablespoon of Maple Syrup

First take and marinate the soy curls in soy sauce, pineapple juice, & maple syrup for around 30 minutes or 1 hour. Then start to prepare your skewers by alternating the veggies and the soy curls. Once these are done grill on a hot grill and serve with any leftover sauce or your favorite sauce.

Hawaiian Sweet Potatoes

6 Sweet Potatoes peeled and cut into 1 inch pieces

1 Cup Coconut Milk (you may need more depending on the consistency of the potatoes)

1 Cup Pineapple (if you use canned save the juice)

¼ Cup Pineapple Juice

¼ Cup Coconut Flakes

2 Tablespoons of Earth Balance

Salt And Pepper To Taste

First take the peeled sweet potatoes and steam them or boil them in water until a fork can go through them. Next drain the sweet potatoes and mash them with the rest of the ingredients and serve! These are great even for the holidays!

Taro Root with Tempeh

4 Taro Roots

3 Tablespoon Light Miso Paste

1 Cup Veggie Broth

1 Package of Tempeh Cut Into Small Squares

Salt and Pepper

2 Tablespoons of Soy Sauce

1 Tablespoon of Agave Nectar

Take the taro roots and clean and peel them and cut them into smaller pieces and cook them with all of the rest of the ingredients (except for the tempeh) until soft and then add the tempeh for the last 10 minutes. Serve in a large serving dish for everyone!

BBQ Soy Curls

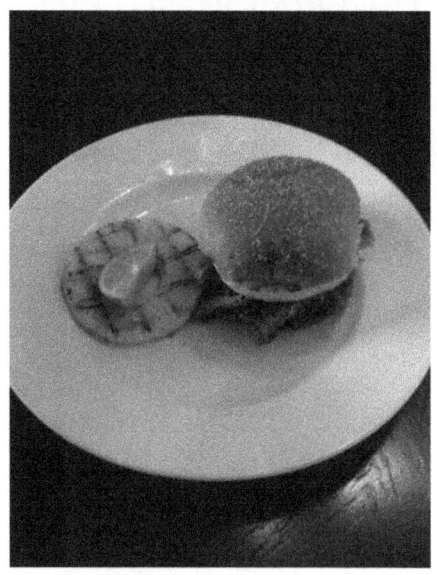

1 Package of Soy Curls (you can also use Tempeh if you like)

1 Bottle of Your Favorite BBQ Sauce (I like Annies Maple BBQ)

Whole Wheat Buns for The Entire Party

Avocado & Pineapple Rings for garnish

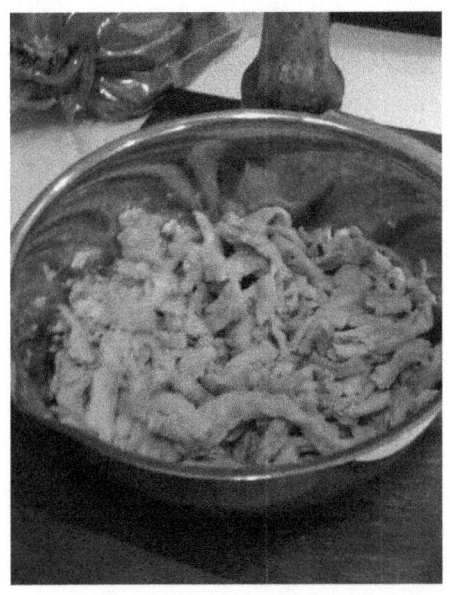

First take and prepare the soy curls as per packages directions. After you drain the soy curls pour the BBQ sauce over the soy curls and soak for an hour or two the longer the better. Sometimes I soak them overnight so that the sauce can soak into the curls. Then take the soy curls and either use a large pan that you can put on your grill and toss them around until good and done or place the curls in a casserole dish and bake at 400 degrees for 25-30 minutes. You can also use a large skillet to brown the soy curls, which only takes 10-15 minutes. Now grill your whole wheat buns and set them on the side so that your guests can make their own BBQ curl sandwich! My favorite thing is to add grilled pineapple rings to them!

Tofu Hawaiian Satay

1 Package of Extra Firm Tofu Drained and Cut Into 1 Inch Squares

1 Cup of the Macadamia Nut Sauce

1 Tablespoon of Curry Powder

Dash of Red Pepper Flakes

First take the cut tofu and soak the pieces in the macadamia nut sauce with the curry powder and red pepper flakes for 30 - 60 minutes. Now thread the tofu onto skewers and grill and serve with leftover macadamia nut sauce.

Grilled Eggplant

1 Large Eggplant

Salt and Pepper

Olive Oil

First take the eggplant and cut into rounds and lay them in a sheet pan and salt the tops and bottoms and let them sit for 30 minutes to let them dry out a bit. Now pepper and olive oil them and grill each side and serve! You can also do this with any other fresh vegetables that available such as bok choy!

Grilled Gardeins with Pineapple

1 Gardein Per Person

1 Pineapple Ring Per Person

Teriyaki Sauce

1 Teaspoon of Grated Ginger

Salt and Pepper

Salt and Pepper the Gardeins and then soak in the teriyaki sauce and grated ginger. Now grill them alongside of the pineapple rings and serve the Gardeins with the pineapple rings on top!

Hawaiian Gardeins

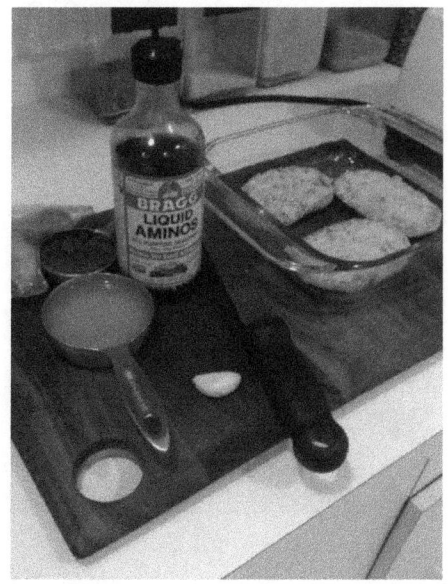

Marinade: This makes enough for 6 Gardeins

1 Cup Pineapple Juice

½ Cup Brown Sugar

2 Tablespoons Soy Sauce

2 Cloves Garlic

1 Teaspoon Ginger

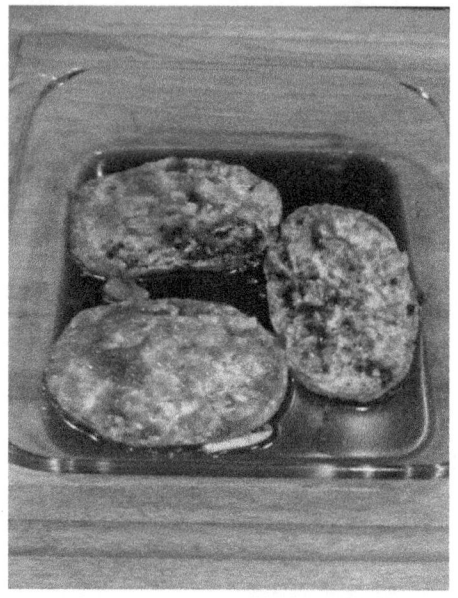

Soak the Gardeins in the Marinade for several hours and then grill! Serve with Hawaiian Rice! You can put the Gardeins in the marinade frozen and let them sit in there to marinate while they de-thaw.

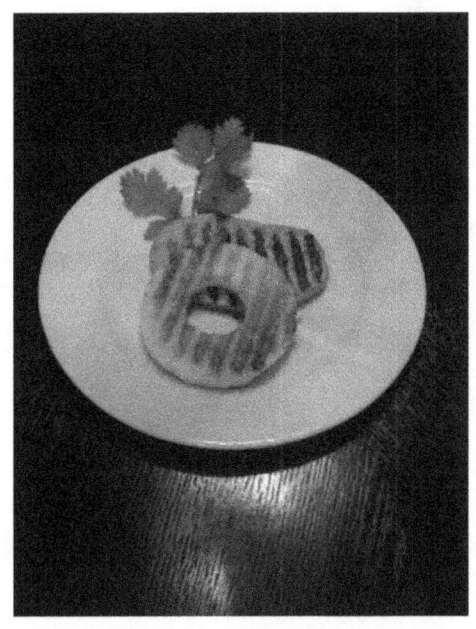

Hawaiian Rum Gardeins

4-6 Gardeins

¼ Cup Rum

¼ Cup Honey

1 Clove of Garlic

2 Tablespoons of Earth Balance

1 Green Bell Pepper Chopped

1 Red Pepper Chopped

1 Can of Drained Pineapple

Melt the butter in the microwave. Place the Gardeins in a baking dish. Mix all of the other ingredients in a bowl and pour over the Gardeins and bake at 400 degrees for 20-25 minutes.

Vegan Hawaiian BBQ Burgers

1 Large Maui Onion Chopped

4 Cloves of Garlic

1 Grated Carrot

3 Tablespoons of Your Favorite BBQ Sauce

1 ½ Cups of Quick Oats

1 Cup Pinto Beans

1 Teaspoon Cumin

2 Teaspoon Chili Powder

2 Teaspoons of Braggs

In a skillet cook the chopped onion, garlic, and carrot. Next mash the pinto beans and add the rest of the ingredients together and form into patties. Grill or fry the vegan burgers in a pan and garnish with avocado & pineapple rings!

Hawaiian Macaroni Salad

1 Large Bag of Elbow Macaroni

1 Cup Vegenaise

2 Teaspoons of Yellow Mustard

1 Tablespoon of Brown Sugar

1 Teaspoon of White Vinegar

2 Stalks of Celery

½ Maui Onion

1 Carrot Grated

Salt and Pepper

Cook the Macaroni as per package. Next chop the celery and onion into small slices. Mix the rest of the ingredients in a bowl and add the cooked and COOLED macaroni and stir well but be careful to not break the macaroni up. Chill and serve!

Hawaiian Desserts

Haupia

Vanilla Haupia

Pineapple Haupia

Frozen Cherry & Pineapple Pie

Coconut Bars

Coconut Ice Cream

Mango Ice Cream

Pineapple & Ginger Ice Cream

Creamy Pineapple Pie

Pineapple Cheesecake

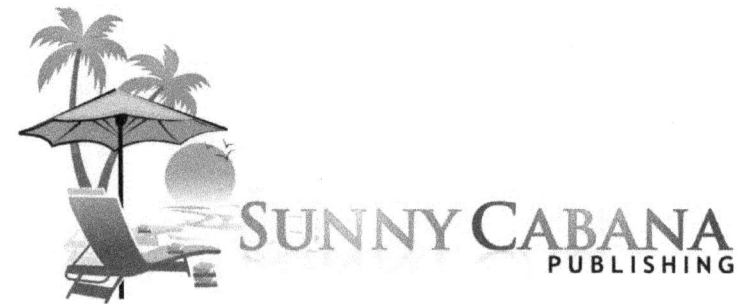

Hawaiian Desserts

Haupia

*This is a pudding

2 Cups of Coconut Milk

1 Cup of Sugar

3 Tablespoons of Agar-Agar Powder

1 Teaspoon of salt

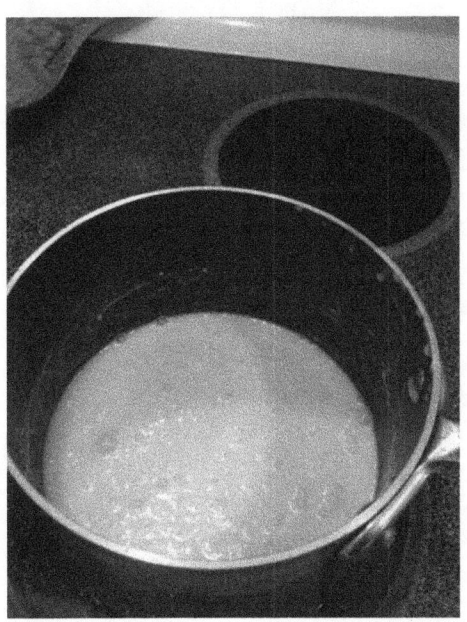

Take all of the ingredients and heat in a sauce pan on the stove until it becomes thick. Don't let it get too hot and you may need to add more arrowroot depending upon the thickness you would like. When that is done pour into a pan and chill to serve for later.

Vanilla Haupia

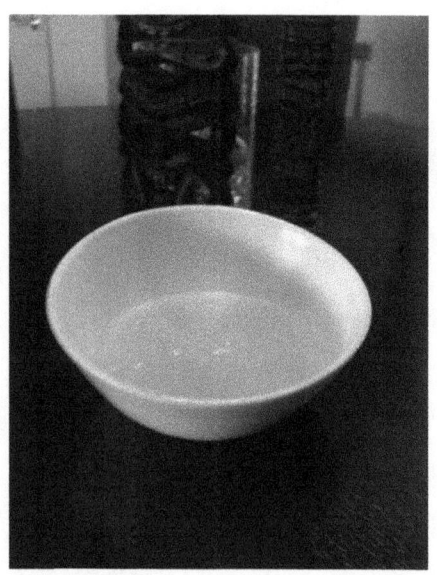

The same as above but just add 1 Fresh Vanilla Bean or vanilla extract to the ingredients! Yum!

Pineapple Haupia

Use the same ingredients but add 1/2 Cup of chopped pineapple to the mix and add an extra tablespoon of agar-agar powder and cook until firm.

Vegan Rum Cake

2 Cups Flour

1 ½ Cups of Sugar

4 Teaspoon Baking Powder

1 Teaspoon salt

½ Cup Earth Balance

½ Cup Canola Oil

1 Package of Vegan Vanilla Powder instant pudding

½ Cup of Rum

1 Teaspoon of Vanilla or a Vanilla Bean Added Is Much Better

½ Cup Almond Milk

4 Teaspoon of Ener-G Egg Replacer

Take all dry ingredients and mix in a separate bowl and then mix all the wet ingredients in another bowl and then blend them together and place in a greased Bundt cake pan and bake for 50 minutes in a 325 degree oven. Serve with vegan whip if you like of grilled pineapple slices!

Frozen Cherry & Pineapple Pie

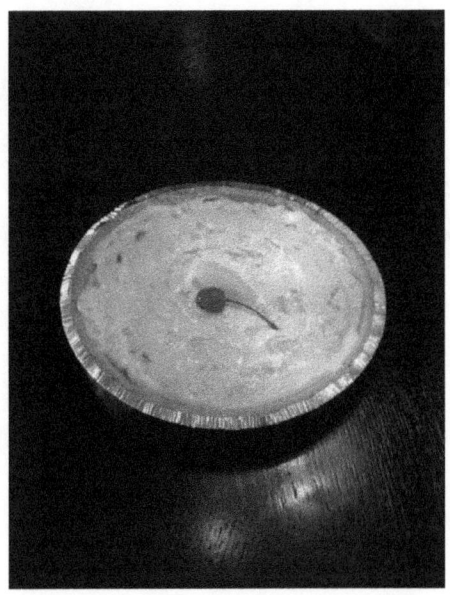

1 Vegan Graham Cracker Pie Crust

1 Large Container of Vegan Whip or two cups of spray whip

1 8 oz Package of Vegan Cream Cheese

1/3 Cup Powdered Sugar

1 Small Can of Drained Pineapple Chunks

½ Cup of Chopped Red Maraschino Cherries

Mix the vegan whip, vegan cream cheese, together until fluffy. Next add the cherries and pineapple and fill up the pie shell and freeze for later!

Coconut Bars

1 Can Coconut Milk

2/3 Cup Brown Sugar

2 Cups Vegan Graham Cracker Crumbs

½ Cup Earth Balance

2 Tablespoons of Sugar

2 Cups of Coconut Flakes

1 Cup Macadamia Nuts

In a saucepan take the coconut milk and brown sugar and heat for around 10 minutes until mixture is mixed well. Next take a pan that is 12x12 and place parchment paper in the bottom of the pan. Now take the graham cracker crumbs, melted earth balance, and the 2 tablespoons of regular sugar and press into the pan. Now pour the coconut mixture on the graham cracker crumbs. The last thing is to take the coconut and place on a baking sheet for a few minutes to brown in a bit and then place that on the top along with the chopped macadamia nuts and make sure everything is pressed together and bake at 350 degrees for 30 minutes or until golden brown.

Coconut Ice Cream

1 Cup Soaked Macadamia nuts or cashews

1 Cup Water

2/3 Cup o Agave Nectar

½ Teaspoon of Vanilla

1 Cup Almond Milk

1 Frozen Banana

½ Cup Coconut Shreds

Pinch of Salt

You will need an ice cream maker for this! Make sure that the ice cream bowl is frozen. Mix all ingredients (except for the coconut) in a high speed mixer and blend until smooth. Now add the coconut flakes and pour into the ice cream maker and mix to the required specifications of the machine. Take the ice cream out of the mixer when done and freeze if it's not quite frozen enough for a couple of hours or you can eat it right way it is but for a party it is easier to make several flavors ahead of time.

Mango Ice Cream

1 Can of Coconut Milk

1 Large Mango Peeled and chopped into small pieces

½ Cup Sugar

1 Teaspoon of Vanilla Extract

Mix all ingredients in a high speed blender and then freeze the mixer for 2 hours and then pour into an ice cream maker and make ice cream and then either freeze or serve right away.

Pineapple & Ginger Ice Cream

1 Cup of Pineapple Chunks

1 Can of Coconut Milk

½ Cup of Brown Sugar

1 Small toe of Ginger Grated

If you can find some crystallized ginger pieces these work well to add to the mixture! (About ¼ Cup)

Mix all ingredients in a high speed blender, add the crystallized ginger, and then freeze this mixture for 2 hours to cool it off. Now add it to the ice cream maker.

Creamy Pineapple Pie

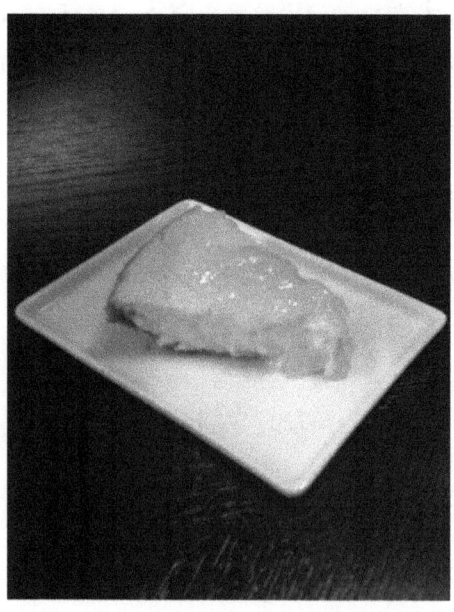

1 Graham Cracker Crust

1 Package of Silken Tofu

1 Container of Tofutti Cream Cheese or Any Other Brand of Vegan Cream Cheese That You Like

1 Cup Sugar

1 Tablespoon of Lime Juice

½ Teaspoon of Vanilla Extract

¾ Cup Pineapple in its Juice

1 Heaping Spoonful of Arrowroot

Topping:

½ Cup Pineapple in its Juice

¼ Cup of Sugar

1 Teaspoon of Arrowroot

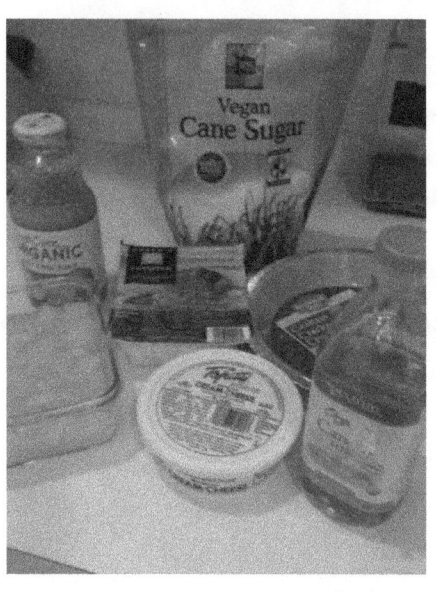

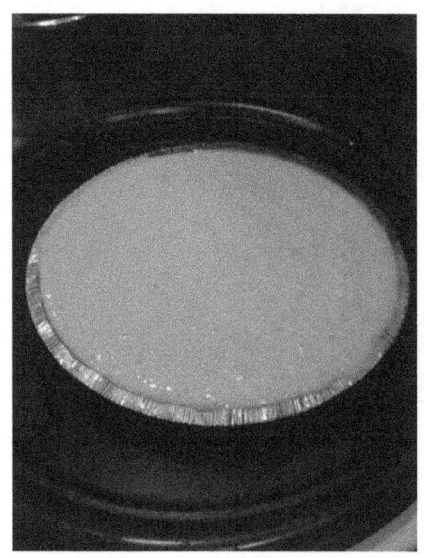

Take all the ingredients except the shell and mix in a high speed blender until smooth. Pour ingredients in the shell and bake at 355 degrees for 55 minutes. Cool pie for an hour and then refrigerate for a couple of hours. You could refrigerate the night before your party! If you want you can garnish the cheesecake right before serving with either chopped pineapple or grilled pineapple rings if you like.

I prefer to make a sauce for the top. Take and mix all of the topping ingredients and cook in a saucepan until thick. Top the cheesecake right before serving.

Pineapple Cheesecake

2 Cups Shredded Coconut

½ Cup Earth Balance

2 Teaspoons of Arrowroot

1 Containers of Tofutti Cream Cheese or Another Vegan brand

1 Cup of Sugar

1 Cup of Pineapple without the Juice

1 Teaspoon Vanilla

To Make the Crust Take a saucepan and melt the earth balance, add the coconut, and only 1 teaspoon of the arrowroot powder. Heat that until it thickens a bit. Now take a lined or greased pan and press this mixture into it to form a crust. Once this is done bake just the crust in a 375 degree oven for 15-20 minutes or until just lightly browned.

Now for the filling: Take the rest of the ingredients and mix in a high speed blender until smooth and pour onto the crust. Bake the pie at 350 degrees for 45 minutes. Cool the pie completely for at least an hour and then refrigerate. You can top the pie when done with crushed pineapple just before serving.

Helpful Tiki Websites

www.Halaukalama.com A Denver based company that has two locations for learning hula dance classes.

www.mele.com This is a super cool website! They list hula schools all over the world.

www.ipolynesia.com

www.TikiMagazine.com

www.Konakai.com This is a very cool tiki shop that has all kinds of items for your next tiki party!

www.ebay.com This site you can use in order to gather your cool tiki attire, glasses, tiki masks or anything else you can think of for your tiki party. It's also nice because you can gather vintage tiki wares for a more authentic tiki look!

www.amazon.com This is a great site for gathering umbrellas for drinks and other cool party favors.

www.youtube.com This is a great site for gathering information on some great tiki groups or great Hawaiian groups!

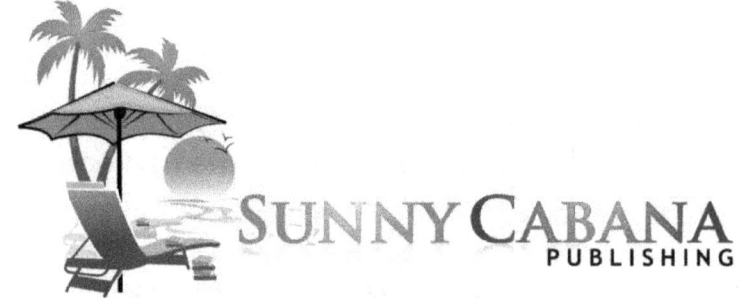

Must Have Tiki Music

www.tikiroom.com This is a great website that lists some great music you can purchase for your next tiki party!

Some Hawaiian music artists that I like are Izrael Kamakawiwo'ole, Zee Ari, Henry Kapono, Don Ho, Alfred Apaka (he does the famous Hukilau song), Sean Na'auao, Keoki Kahumoku (does a great job with the slide guitar) and there are so many more great Hawaiian music artists that you should check out!

Below is a list musical artists that are considered the best at shaping the tiki musical scene but really it all depends on your likes and dislikes. You can also check out you tube for other artists you may like even better.

- ❖ Martin Denny created the "Exotica" sound popular in the 1950s and 1960s that mixed Latin rhythms with a little piano, a little background echo and maybe a few bird calls along with large bongo drum and marimbas. Denny most popular hit is called "Quiet Village" in 1958. It's great music from one of the finest lounge acts in American history.

- The Smokin' Menehunes are number two because of their more traditional Hawaiian music. But they are a Southern California group that plays Hawaiian music with a large bass, steel guitar, and lyrics about the Waikiki sands and the swaying palms. I really like their upbeat sounds!
- Arthur Lyman is another stalwart of the Exotica era, a Hawaiian born vibraphone player that made a career out of the Polynesian sound. Lyman billed himself as the "King of Lounge Music." We believe his talents are worthy of being re-introduced as a member of the royalty in the realm of Tiki bar music. He does a great rendition of Yellow Bird! I love that song!
- Clouseaux" is a contemporary group making some noise on the commercial Tiki lounge circuit with their sound that has solid

percussions with loud monkey sounds.
- ❖ Sonny Chillingworth is a master of the Hawaiian slack-key guitar, a style of open tuning playing that originated in the Islands. He recorded principally Polynesian tunes but was capable of many types of finger picking styles. He also talks about how he plays the slack key guitar with a needle and thread! It's a pretty cool story that he tells about his grandfather not being allowed to be seen with his grandmother so his grandfather would take thread and tie it to her window at night and have a needle on the other end that would bounce off the guitar strings and the music would vibrate to her window at night.
- ❖ Yma Sumac was a Peruvian soprano with an extraordinary vocal range that became a popular performer and recording artist in the 1950s and 1960s. Her music merged South American and horn playing rhythms but her voice was the remarkable.

- Gabby Pahinui was a Hawaiian pedal steel and slack key guitar master that had a career spanning four decades beginning in the 1930s as a poor Hawaiian kid playing in club bands. In the 1970s he was a key player in the "Hawaiian Renaissance" that saw many recording artists returning to traditional Hawaiian styles and modernizing them for music that is a perfect fit for a Tiki bar gathering today. His sounds are what you think of for tiki music it's soothing and I would definitely try to find his music to play at my next tiki party!
- Les Baxter was an accomplished American composer, arranger and pianist who worked as a producer and worked on scored films such as the documentary Tanga Tika (1953) and recorded his own material. In the 1970s he was recognized as one of the principal creators of the Exotica sound. His music is an orchestrated version of the genre. It has a very jazzy sound!
- Don Tiki is a couple of Hawaiian musicians who produce Tiki concept

albums that not only honor the tradition of Exotica but bring it into the present. Their music is a top notch mix of Polynesian sounds, quality vocals and backup from a great different mix of Hawaiian musicians and hula girls!
- ❖ Another great Hawaiian musical artist is Aunty Genoa Keawe. She has crazy high pitch sounds (falsetto). Her music is truly awesome! It's so unique that you almost can't stop listening.

Music does make the mood so make sure that you have the type of music that both you and your friends will like for your tiki party. Either way it will be fun!

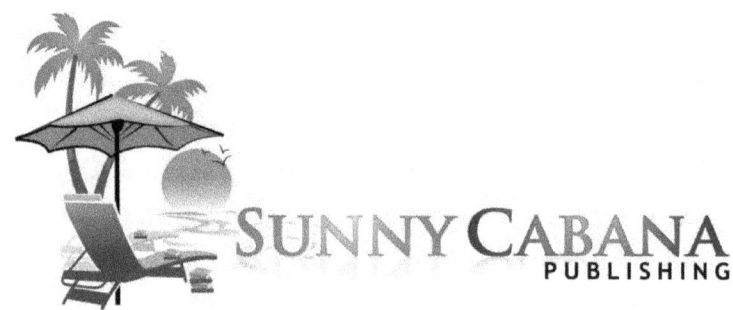

Hawaiian Sayings for Your Party

Aloha: Hi or Good Bye Love

Hele Mei Hoohiwahiwa: Come celebrate

La Hanau: Birthday

Hau`oli la Hanau Happy Birthday

Hale: Home or building

Kai: Sea

Pono: Excellent

Popo: Appetizers

Ono: Deliscious

Nui: Important/Big

A hui hou kakou: Until we meet again

Aloha kakahiaka: Good morning

Aloha `auinala: Good afternoon

Aloha ahiahi: Good evening

Aloha `oe: Farewell to you

A'ole pilikia: No problem

Hana Hou!: One more time!

Hau'oli la Ho'omana'o: Happy Anniversary

Hau'oli Makahiki Hou: Happy New Year

Kipa hou mai: Come visit again

Mahalo: Thank you

Mahalo nui loa: Thank you very much

Mele Kalikimaka Merry Christmas

Mau: Forever

Nau wale no: Just for you

'O wai kou inoa?: What is your name?

Pomaika'i: Good Luck

Some Helpful Vegan Websites

www.veganmainstream.com Great for vegan businesses! I was interviewed on this site!

www.vegan.com

www.supervegan.com

www.goveg.com

www.kidbean.com (vegan kid clothing and accessories)

www.vegancoach.com

www.vegansociety.com

www.findaspring.com

www.cosmeticdatabase.com

www.etsy.com This site has particular sellers that have etsyveg next to their items if they support the vegan lifestyle or their products are vegan!

www.vegnews.com This is a great website to help promote your vegan business along with great tips on a vegan diet!

www.veganstore.com They have great vegan white chocolate chips!

www.veganoutreach.org

www.veganpassport.com When you travel you will want to check this website out. *They also have an app for your phone! Yeah!*

www.Barnivore.com This is a cool website that tells you what alcohol is vegan! Awesome!

www.vegtv.com

www.happycow.net

www.quarrygirl.com

www.fatfreevegan.com

www.edenfoods.com

www.planetgreen.com

www.veganproductguide.com

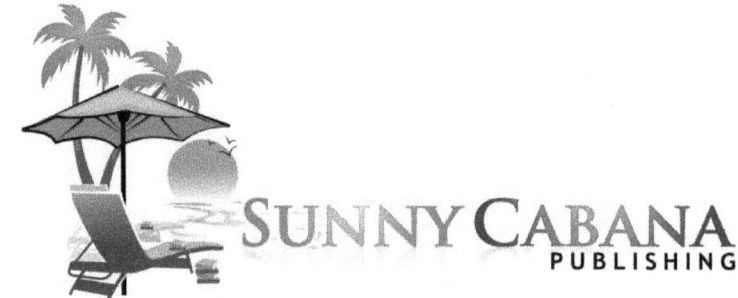

Some Helpful Vegan Phone Apps

Vegan Yum Yum. This app lets you search, view, and organize all your favorite vegan recipes.

VeganXpress. If you are on the go a lot then this app will work for you. Veganxpress lets you see what restaurants and fast food places have vegan fare.

VegScan. This is a great app that you can scan the barcode to check to see if the food product is vegan or vegetarian! So cool!

HappyCow. This is one of my favorites! I love the website and the app! This app lets you have vegan and vegetarian restaurants on the go. There is an interactive map that shows you where the restaurants and stores are located. There is also phone numbers, directions, and their websites. You can also share on facebook & twitter! I big bonus if you find something really great!

WholeFoodsMarket. This is a great app that allows you to search for recipes, with nutritional information, add ingredients to your shopping list, store locator! This is great if you are traveling!

Eden Recipes. This is great for recipes and sharing them on facebook!

Gardein Recipes. I love these things! They are so tasty! This is a great app if you just don't know what goes with a gardein.

Cruelty-Free. This is a great app for shopping animal free!

VegWeb. This app has vegan recipes.

Veggie Passport. This is a great app if you are traveling and you want to explain what you can or cannot eat. You can choose your language (there are lots to choose from) and then chose the message you want to tell the waiter. This is very useful and weighs less than a phrase book.

There are so many apps out there! Plus they change daily! Just keep up to date!

It's the greatest way to keep your diet in check!

Go Vegan. *Over 50 recipes*

Be Vegan

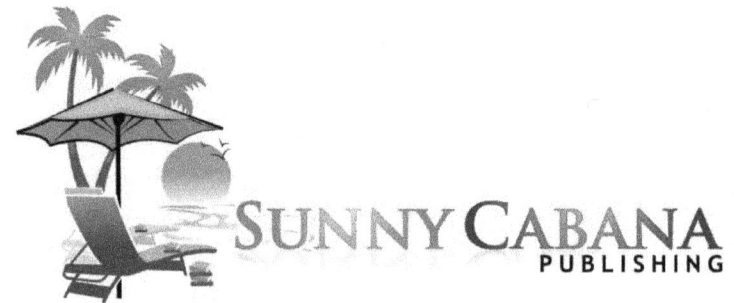

VEGAN COOKINGS CLASSES AND SCHOOLS

CALIFORNIA

Spork Foods
7494 Santa Monica Blvd Ste 302
W Hollywood, CA 90046
www.sporkonline.com

Living Light Culinary Arts Institute
704 N Harrison
Fort Bragg, CA 95437
www.rawfoodchef.com

Bay Area Vegetarians
PO Box 700
Vallejo, CA 94590-0069
www.bayareaveg.org

The New School of Cooking
8690 Washington Blvd
Culver City, CA 90232
310-842-9702
www.newschoolofcooking.com

Hip Cooks
642 Moulton Ave
Los Angeles, CA 90031
323-222-3663
www.hipcooks.com
They are also located in Portland, OR, Seattle, WA, East and West LA.

HAWAAII

Vegan Fusion
www.veganfusion.com
PO Box 1119
Kapaa, HI 96746

NEW YORK

Natural Gourmet Institute for Health & Culinary Arts
48 W 21st St 2nd Floor
New York, NY 10010
212-645-5170
www.naturalgourmetinstitute.com

NORTH CAROLINA

Lenoresnatural.com
Lenore Baum
164 Ox Creek Rd
Weaverville, NC 28787
828-645-1412

VIRGINIA

Mimi Clarks Vegan Cooking Classes
9302 Hallston Ct
Fairfax Station, VA 22039
703-643-2713
www.veggourmet.wordpress.com

TEXAS
The Natural Epicurean Academy of Culinary Arts
1700 S Lamar Blvd
Austin, TX 78704
512-476-2276
www.naturalepicurean.com

CANADA

Live Nutrition Cooking School
5 Kitsilano Crescent
Richmond Hill
Ontario, L4C 5A4
905-884-9112
www.livenutritionschool.com

The Vegan Vegetarian Cooking School
3988 Galloway Frt Rd
Elko, BC V0B 1J0
250-529-7750

ENGLAND

Cordon Vert Vegetarian Cookery School
Parkdale
Dunham Rd
Altrinchaum
Cheshire, England
01619252014
www.cordonvert.co.uk
(They are a vegetarian school but they make exceptions for vegan)

About the Author

B.S. in Physical Anthropology, Minor in Business, and Art Institute of Fort Lauderdale Culinary Arts Degree.

Advocate for organic, vegetarian, vegan, and raw food diets. I have been a vegetarian/vegan/raw foodist for over 20 years. Owner of Sunny Cabana Publishing, L.L.C. and a published author of living foods and raw food recipe books for Recipes 4 Raw Food, The Vivacious Vegan, & The Vivacious Vegan Desserts.

Have several websites to help people who are interested in healthy eating www.Recipes4RawFood.com, and www.RawFoodForToday.com.

Owner of www.RawFoodsAssociation.com and www.SunnyCabanaPublishing.com

Follow me on Facebook: facebook.com/sunnycabanapublishing

Email: SunnyCabanaPublishing@gmail.com

Or TheVivaciousVegan@gmail.com

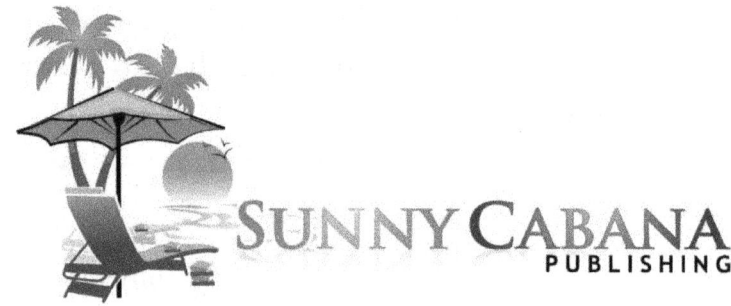

Index

A
Agave Nectar Page 32, 64, 91, 112
Appetizers Page 5, 57, 59
Avocados Page 58, 79, 80, 81, 82, 93, 101

B

Bananas Page 34, 39, 53, 54, 112
Boat Drinks Page 5, 39, 41
Burgers Page

C
Carrots Page 87
Celery Page 83, 101
Cheesecake Page 103, 117
Cilantro Page 61, 62, 65, 76, 81, 88
Coconut Page 13, 23, 28, 29, 34, 44, 50, 54, 57, 66, 67, 68, 69, 71, 72, 74, 83, 90, 103, 105, 110, 111, 112, 113, 117, 118
Cucumbers Page 76, 79, 80, 81

D

Desserts Page 103, 105

E

F

G

Garlic Page 61, 77, 79, 97, 99, 100, 101
Guava Page 23, 25, 32, 33, 39, 44, 48, 49, 50, 51
Ginger Page 57, 63, 64, 96, 98, 103, 113, 114

H

Hawaiian Page 5, 10, 11, 12, 13, 20, 50, 79, 83, 87, 88, 89, 90, 94, 97, 98, 99, 100, 103, 105, 121-125, 127

I

Ice Cream Page 103, 111, 112, 113, 114

J

K

Kiwi Page 34, 35

L

Lemon Page 31, 46, 52
Limes Page 23, 31, 75, 77, 79

M

Macadamia Nuts Page 25, 36, 57, 65, 66, 67, 71, 72, 74, 75, 87, 94, 95, 110, 111
Main Courses Page 85, 87
Mangoes Page 25, 35, 39, 55, 57, 60, 76, 103, 113
Mint Page 23, 25, 28, 31, 37, 49
Music Page

N

O

Orange Page 25, 28, 29, 30, 31, 32, 33, 35, 46, 47, 48, 51, 63

P

Papaya Page 25, 30, 34, 52, 76, 82
Phone Apps Page 131
Pineapple Page 23, 27, 28, 33, 34, 47, 48, 49, 50, 51, 52, 57, 58, 62, 65, 73, 74, 75, 78, 83, 85, 87, 89, 90, 94, 96, 97, 100, 101, 103, 107-118
Pudding Page 105, 108

Q

R

Rice Page 85, 87

Rum Page 8, 10, 23, 36, 39, 41, 44, 45, 46, 47, 48, 49, 50, 75, 99, 107

S

Soy Sauce Page 64, 68, 76, 87, 89, 91, 97
Strawberries Page 25, 29, 78
Sweet Potato Page 85, 90, 91

T

Tempeh Page 57, 70, 85, 89, 91, 92
Teriyaki Sauce Page 57, 64, 70, 88, 96
Tofu Page 57, 63, 64, 65, 66, 67, 68, 69, 72, 85, 87, 94, 95, 115
Tomatoes Page 89

U

V

Vegan Schools Page 137

W

Watermelon Page 78

X, Y, Z

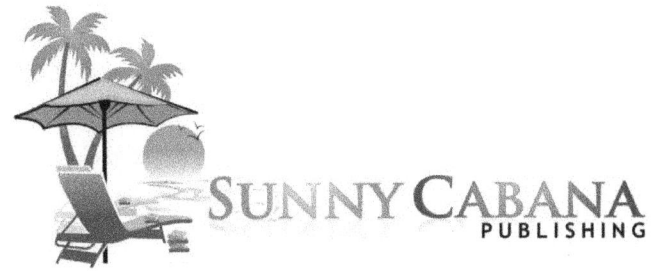

The Vivacious Vegan Desserts

$14.95

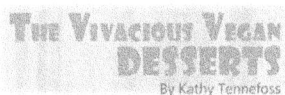

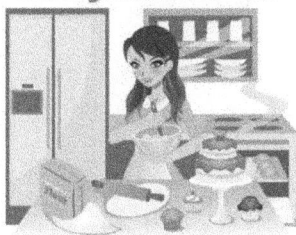

80 Awesome Raw Food Recipes You Can't Live Without $14.95

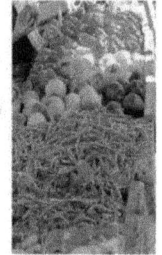

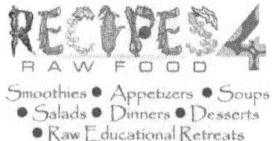
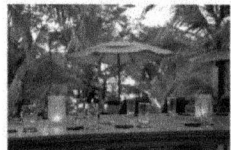

Awesome Raw Food Guide $15.95

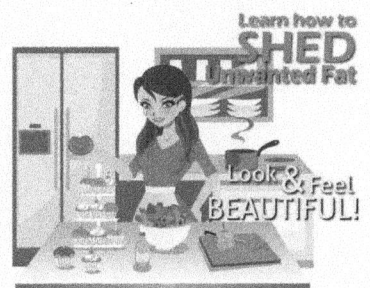

The Vivacious Vegan $13.95

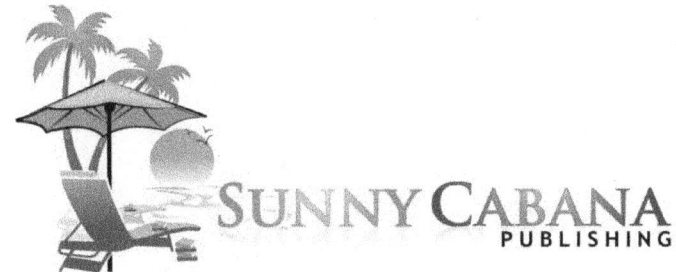

www.SunnyCabanaPublishing.com

SunnyCabanaPublishing@gmail.com

www.ingramcontent.com/pod-product-compliance
Lightning Source LLC
LaVergne TN
LVHW011422080426
835512LV00005B/218